Taming
Your Pain

by

Disclaimer

The use of any or all of these tools, techniques, exercises, movements, and/or ideas are only opinions and suggestions. You know and are aware of your body and your own limitations. None of this material is intended to cause pain and/or harm; if pain occurs it is the result of your actions and you accept full responsibility for the outcome. You will hold Cheryl Weekes and/or any associates harmless of any wrong doing through means of these materials presented. Your participation in any part of this course is at your own free will; you assume complete responsibility; and you are fully accountable. You should consult your physician before attempting any or all of this program. The outcomes of using any of the information contained in this book are generally expected results.

Table of Contents

Forward

The mainstream model of health care has the majority of people believing their health is taken care of for them. When we feel sick we simply go to the doctors, preferably ones with a white coats and a stethoscopes around their collar, where they find a name that best describes our particular symptoms and confidently prescribes a solution. Inevitably, this solution comes in a form of a pill. We take the pill; the symptoms abate; and we move on with our lives.

The trouble with this convenient model is it only hides the symptoms and will most likely create new ones. This only addresses the physical aspect of our bodies which now has to recover from the toxic chemicals we just consumed! We forget that the body is a self-healing organism and despite what we put into it, it will recover from most ailments on its own. This model has been sufficient for handling emergencies and acute situation but has failed when it comes to chronic, long-term illnesses such as arthritis, allergies, chronic fatigue, depression, fibromyalgia, and neuropathy. Again these diagnoses are just names assigned to a group of symptoms and have no way of addressing the cause of these symptoms. *It is time to wake from this illusion and take our bodies and our health into our own hands.*

Since this is new territory for most people, *this book is the perfect tool* to open your mind to what I believe is the "new frontier" in health care today. If we want to get to the true cause of our ailments, we must consider the other 75% of ourselves, not just the physical part but the mental, emotional, and spiritual aspects as well. When we experience a physical trauma it becomes rooted in our emotional body. If the trauma was from a car accident, then you may experience anxiety every time you get into a car. If this emotional stress is never neutralized, the anxiety may continue to grow until you find yourself too afraid to set foot in a car again.

Likewise, emotional traumas you experience throughout your life express themselves through the physical body. Anyone can see when someone is sad or happy because it is revealed in how they express it. Now image all the negative emotional traumas you have experienced throughout your lifetime and how they might relate to the pain or illness you might be experiencing today.

As you practice the exercises in this book, you will discover that many memories will surface that you have hidden from yourself! Memories that may have been too painful for you to deal with when they occurred so your mind conveniently tucked them away until you were ready. *Now is the TIME!* The only way out is through.

The information and exercises awaiting you on the following pages provide you with the tools necessary to begin your journey of self-healing AND self-discovery. You will be able to reclaim your health and decide for yourself what course of action to take when you do seek professional help and not to blindly follow them based on fear and lack of knowledge.

Stay open minded to look at your life choices in a new light and as you do, you will discover the true experience of joy and gratitude for every precious moment we receive in this life.

I am confident that you are willing, ready, and able to move forward and *take your well being into your own hands.* So be adventurous and step into this great journey of self-care, self-health. This is just the beginning....

Steven P. Matthewson, D.C.
Bellevue Natural Health
Washington

Introduction

Most people go around a-hoping and a-wishing, by some magical event, something good will happen to them or they'll wake up one morning and all their pain will be gone and they will live happily ever after.

Sorry, if that applies to you - that's not going to happen. Yes miracles do happen but not by some magical potion or a wand waved over you.

The only true thing that is going to make you happy is having the experience, on a regular basis, that you are making progress in your life. Right?

Having or getting something is not going to make you happy either. It's doing things that will create happiness. You must feel progression in a positive direction. And this doesn't *just* happen - it only happens when you take control of the direction and action.

The first step is to have a path with clearly defined actions. That's what this book can offer you. This 10-treatment course will present some tools for you to implement into your daily routine that will propel and pull (not push) you 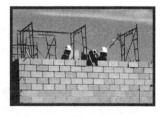 towards a more positive lifestyle and ultimately lower your pain. It will lay a foundation, an understanding of concepts that may be familiar to some of you and totally new to others.

According to Brain Statistics, there are 116 million Americans suffering from chronic pain. Out of those 116 million, only 14% of the people will take action beyond the basic treatment program prescribed by their doctors. In other words, only 1 out of 7 people will seek alternative healing options once they finish a conventional medical program. That means 86% of the people who suffer great pain either revert back to their old "habit" patterns; simply give up because they didn't see any improvement with their current treatment program; and/or believe there is nothing more that can be done.

Wow - 86% of sufferers are still in chronic pain and will only get worse with time.

Thank goodness that's not you. You are among the **14% who are to be applauded for reading this** book. That means you are not satisfied and/or will not accept being in pain for the rest of your life. Yahooooooooo - you are willing and able to take action to lower your pain levels and start living again.

According to Tony Robbins, "Ultimately, if you are going to have lasting change in anything, you must raise your standards." So are you willing to do a few things that may seem a bit odd at first to raise your standards in order to lower your pain? Are you willing to make it a "must" in your life instead of a "should"?

I have faith in you - I know *you are willing* to have an open attitude towards something that might s-t-r-e-t-c-h you a bit because, after all, you are part of the 14 percentile and - - - - - -
you are definitely a cut above the norm.

I will talk more about standards later so for now I want to give you some benefits that this course can give you if you are consistent, disciplined, and willing to follow through with the homework.

You could easily read this book cover to cover and say OK, I've read it. But it won't be of much good to you. It is when you actually build the layers on a solid foundation that you will start seeing results. And isn't that what we all want - positive results?

So, I'm assuming that your results thus far have not been up to your standards - let's do something about that together - right now. It's hard to quantify the benefits you will receive from this course. It depends on how much you embrace the assignments and concepts. Each person's pain is their own journey. This book can only present the information and the rest is up to you. Like that old saying, "You can bring the horse to the trough but you can't make it drink the water." Whether you decide to drink the water or not is completely up to you.

Because I am so excited with my results using these methods, I want to gift you **ALL** the information that has helped me. Several mentors and colleagues of mine have said, "No-no, save some stuff for your next book". But if I withheld any information I would feel like I was cheating you. So yes, there's a lot of information and it all fits together like a jigsaw puzzle to produce the whole picture. My wish for you is to have a similar experience as I; I want you to feel good again; I want you to be happy again; I want you to start living a productive and contributing lifestyle that your pain has robbed you from up to this point.

One of my biggest ahas was when I realized that if happiness is a choice, then unhappiness is a choice also. My desire for you is to offer you a choice - a choice that perhaps you didn't know existed until now.

This book is not about being your friend. I don't care about how you injured yourself or how someone else is to blame. That may be a bit uncaring and callus but I'm here to *help you lower your pain.* I won't get down into the ditch of "woe-is-me" to wallow around in the mud with you and join you in your pain. I've spent too much time in my own muck and mire ditch. I will not go backwards now that I've worked so hard to get healthy again.

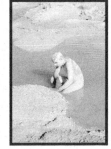

What I will do is stand firmly on the edge of your ditch and throw

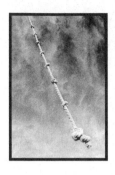 a rope over the edge that is tied securely around my waist. Along the length of this rope are tied knots. Each knot is a set of tools and/or actions methodically organized to build on top of the other. It is up to you to grab the end of this rope and hang on as you take one step at a time out of the ditch. It was you who dug your ditch and now it is time for you to get yourself out.

Each one of us has our own quests and the journey is a personal one, however, my desire is that you use these tools and techniques to help guide you to your own healing.

In Deborah King's book, *Truth Heals: What you hide can hurt you,* she states, "Our wounds always lead us on quests - consciously or unconsciously - toward healing."

Again, in no manner what so ever is my intention to hint at or to convey any perception that I am a miracle worker or that what I offer in this book will heal or cure you. You are your own healer if you believe it. The only thing I will do is hold a place for you in my heart, sincerely offer you what has helped me, and truly believe in your ability to start **lowering your pain levels so you can tame the beast called peripheral neuropathy.**

Who Am I?

That's a great question. And further more, why do I feel qualified to talk to you about this subject?

I am someone just like you who has gone through "hell" and back several times. I mean several times because I'm a slow learner - well, maybe a better way to say it is that I'm a very stubborn learner. This is why...

I grew up with a military-lifer father. To be more specific, a drill sergeant who treated me as a son instead of a daughter. I was taught (drilled) that whenever you fell down, you picked yourself up by the boot straps, dusted yourself off, pushed through the pain, and kept going. Well, that's exactly what I did over 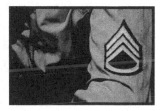 and over again throughout my lifetime - I was tough.

Then one day I heard the word that puts fear in us...Cancer! I felt the walls simply fade away as I sat in the doctor's office while he read his report. Without looking at me he continued, "We need to schedule radiation and chemotherapy as soon as possible." I sat glued to my chair for what seemed an eternity before I could speak. "No - No - No! I won't do it!" I screamed back. I'm sure the doctor was not used to someone questioning his treatment program since he washed his hands of me. Instead of conventional treatment I opted for changing my diet and daily routine. And guess what - it worked because I'm still here after 30 years.

In 2008 my husband was offered a fantastic job in Maryland so within a month we left our home in Washington State. Our son went with us but we left behind two daughters, my business, and the rest of my family and friends. Thank goodness we became acquainted with some really nice people in our new neighborhood but during the next five years I tip-toed in "hell".

My mother became very ill so I was flying across country to co-care for her on hospice with COPD, along with my father who had Alzheimer's. Then my father-in-law in Tucson developed pancreatic cancer so I co-cared for him also. Within three years they all passed. I was so caught up in taking care of my loved 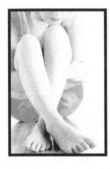 ones that I didn't realize I was putting every-one's health above my own.

I started having pain in my feet and legs but attributed it to shin-splits because I was walking 2 to 5 miles a day just to keep my sanity. The more the pain continued to escalate, the more I was forcing myself to "push through it" just as I was taught.

Now I believe in God and I agree with Oprah when she says that when God wants to get your attention He first **whispers** in your ear, then He **nudges** your shoulder. If that doesn't get your attention, next comes a **thump** on the head. And then comes the **shove**.

The **whisper**:
The pain in my feet and legs had now risen to 24/7 of burning pins and needles. I wasn't sleeping at night because that's when I felt the pain the most and it hurt just to have the bed sheets touch my feet so I started using a fan to help cool them through the night.

The **nudge**:
Since my husband and I were right in the middle of remodeling our house which we were doing most of the work ourselves, I ignored the whisper and kept "dusting myself off". I started experiencing the feeling of electrical shocks along with a buzzing sensation throughout my body including my face and lips - it felt like I had stuck my finger into the wall socket. Then I passed a

kidney stone - talk about pain - it was worse than having a baby!!!

The *thump*:

Because my feet had become so swollen and painful I couldn't wear shoes - only flip flops and it was garbage day - in January - in Maryland. Well I took two steps and down I went flat on my back onto the ice. I was able to right myself but had to crawl on my hands and knees back into the house. I started having migraine headaches on a daily basis and the fall had created a new pain in my hip - like a red-hot poker being stabbed into the joint. So now I was taking 6 to 8 ibuprofens every 3 to 4 hours to try to numb the pain.

Then came a 2nd and 3rd thump - 2 more kidney stones...
Still not listening.

The *shove*:

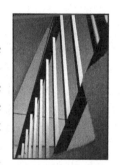

On one of my sleepless nights I noticed that the downstairs light was left on. Well all I remember was taking one step and falling down the stairs. Now, I'm not saying that God shoved me down those stairs - what I'm saying is I couldn't feel the floor under my feet and down I went. It certainly got my attention this time. Thank goodness the only additional injury I incurred was a dislocated shoulder (on top of more injury to my hip, back, feet, and legs). I started popping more and more pain pills until I ended up back in the hospital emergency room with gastritis.

OK, now I'm listening!

Over the next 6 months I spent 10s of thousands of dollars seeing one specialist after another. I was poked and prodded from one end to the other and was left being told that my pain was either in my head (you've got to be kidding me - why would I make this up!) or there was nothing that they could do for me; that I would just have to live with it. One neurologist, in particular, walked me to a closet, opened the door where there were several boxes of pills, reached in grabbing handfuls and filled a plastic bag full of samples. His comment to me was, " Try these and see if anything helps." No information - no side affect warnings - nothing! I refused his "gift" and sought another doctor.

In April of 2012, my husband returned from work one day beaming from ear to ear. He was offered his dream job back in Washington State so I remained in MD for the next four months to sell our house. Three hours after signing the closing papers I was on a flight to Fort Lauderdale, FL. because our son (23 years old) was diagnosed with a very rare form of lung cancer. The immediate family joined me and I took care of him. I was there when he gasped, choked, and took his last breath. I thought I had experienced death before but no one should have to watch their child die. I knew I had to be strong because the rest of the family was falling apart - they were counting on me. So ... once again, I buried my pain and my feelings so I could take care of all the details.

When I arrived back home in Washington State, my house was full of boxes because obviously, I wasn't there when all of our belongings were delivered. I went into robot mode - I had one month to make all the arrangements for our son's memorial which meant out-of-town guests staying at our house for 4 days. No time to grieve or address my own health issues - I had to unpack, clean, arrange furniture, wash dishes, do laundry, make beds, buy groceries, cook, etc. Well, you get the picture.

That whole month was a blur and then the day after the memorial it happened...............

BOOM!!!

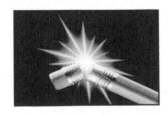

My pain, both physical and emotional, literally picked me up, threw me down on the floor, put its foot on me and held me 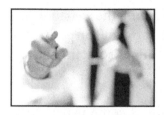 down. It was as if it had a life of its own. I could actually feel a finger pointing down at me and it was screaming at me with such anger, "YOU WILL NOT GET UP. YOU WILL NOT IGNORE ME. YOU ARE MINE. I OWN YOU!!!"

And that was that - I couldn't get up - I had nothing left in me. I was no longer in control of my pain, it was in control of me.

So I know your pain - I know how it feels when your life becomes your pain; when nothing else matters but your pain. That's all you can think about day and night because that's all you feel - pain - pain - and more pain!

I was a broken woman who could no longer pull myself up by my bootstraps, dust myself off, push through the pain, and keep going. I was done. All the doctors in Maryland couldn't help me and now I was in far, far worse shape than before.

I was packing my feet in ice throughout the day and night, not sleeping at all, and had migraine headaches constantly. I was no longer able to be active. It hurt to sit up; it hurt to lie down; it hurt to do the things I loved like going for walks, hiking in the woods, gardening, or even spending time shopping with my daughters. I didn't even want to talk to anyone (that's a sad day when I don't feel like talking).

I was in dire straits. I was bent over. I shuffled instead of being able to walk normally, and I had to run my hand along the wall to keep my balance. My feet were so swollen that I could only wear flip flops. I had always been such a fighter and now I was getting desperate. Was this all I had to look forward to? Only getting worse instead of better? I cried often.

Then on one of my "clearer" days, I was surfing the web for some hope when I saw an ad for cold laser treatment for peripheral neuropathy. Aha... (a light bulb lit up) - this is something I had not tried so I made an appointment.

Sitting down in the waiting room to fill out some paper work, I placed my ice pack on my feet (I never went anywhere without it). As I looked around, I couldn't believe what I was seeing. The other patients were going from station to station while smiling and talking to each other. I let out a big sigh and realized I was finally in the right place. I immediately signed up for the treatment program and it was the best decision I have ever made since I first started having neuropathy related pain issues.

Was this program an instant miracle? No, it was a process with activities I had to do at the clinic as well as at home. After the first 5 treatments I began to notice some improvement and this continued throughout the sessions.

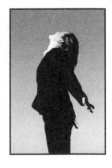

On a pain level scale of 0 (meaning no pain) to 10 (meaning unbearable pain), I had gone from a 10 down to a 5. I was thrilled to say the least. For the first time in 4 years I was able to live a normal life style again. I could think clearly and sleep better (yeah). I was finding joy in my life again. I even was able to meet my daughter in Iceland and go hiking for a week.

The cold laser treatment program literally gave me my life back! But I had hit a plateau and there was nothing more the clinic could do for me. Now don't get me wrong, I will always be indebted to that clinic, however, I was not satisfied to remain at a pain level 5 for the rest of my life - not now, now that I had come this far. So I resumed my normal treatments with Dr. Steve

Matthewson (awesome chiropractor - Bellevue Natural Health) and I started searching for other alternative methods to improve my health and ultimately lower my pain even more. Remember, I'm a fighter and my father taught me well and now I was able to wear "boots" again.

I spent months digging through data and findings. I would use myself as a guinea pig. I wrote down what methods reduced my pain and what didn't. Through trial and error I developed a program that not only lowered my pain but allowed me to function at an even higher level as a healthy, energetic, loving, joyful person again. My husband was so impressed with my transformation that he started doing some of these methods himself with great results and so have many others.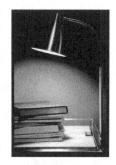

So there you have it .... this is why I feel I am qualified to present this program to you. I'm just like you and since it has worked for me, I am confident it will work for you.

Please keep in mind *I know your pain - I've been there. You are not alone.* Even though there are no wounds, no bandages, no scars, *you are experiencing real pain - it's not in your head and there is something that can be done!*

Have I cured myself? No, I would be lying to make that kind of claim and I won't make that promise for you either. My target is to get to a 0 pain level and I'm still working toward that. Most of the time I'm at a level 1 or 2 and if I have a spike in my pain, it is the result of physically over-doing something or eating sugar.

What I truly believe is that when you integrate this program into your lifestyle, you make it your own. You will start living again in spite of your pain; you will be *taming neuropathy*, just like me.

"Each patient carries his own doctor inside of him. They come to us not knowing the truth. We are at our best when we give the doctor that resides within us a chance to work."

Albert Schweitzer

So Why Aren't Doctors Offering This?

In my opinion, there are several reasons: Most medical professional simply don't know about what I'm going to present to you because this information is not taught in any type of conventional medical schooling.

The few who have heard about it may not believe it can produce positive results. They may consider it to be "alternative" with not enough scientific data to back it by their standards and the American Medical Association.

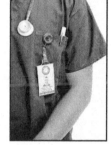

Many professionals may feel they are the only ones, not the patient, qualified to diagnose and treat any condition. Or they may believe that they cannot make money teaching these methods. No drugs to promote so they can get kick-backs from pharmaceutical companies. No service or medical equipment needed in order to charge patients and insurance companies for usage. If patients heal themselves then there's no need for special treatment plans or long-term services.

Please do not misunderstand me, I firmly believe there is a time and place for medical intervention especially in times of crisis and/or emergencies. If I found myself mangled by a car accident, you bet I would want a medical team on my side so I sincerely respect the majority of the individuals in the medical profession who truly care about their patients' well being.

Although it is a slow process, more and more physicians, psychiatrists, therapist, etc. are starting to embrace new ideas and technology but I often question some of the underlying motives of certain institutions that regulate our health care systems by making huge profits from someone's pain and suffering that could easily be alleviated through alternative practices and means.

What I offer in the following pages are my opinions and research. I make no promises or guarantees to the outcomes and results of using the methods presented. Although I'm not alone in this thought area, it is totally up to you to make your own intelligent choices and conclusions.

So

Let's

Get

Started ...

W_{eek} 1
1_{st} K_{not}

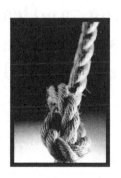

"A wise man should consider that health is the greatest of human blessings, and lear how, by his own thought, to derive from his illness."

Hippocrates

Glorious Day

To me, this is the first step of setting your vibration in a positive direction. It is performed every morning as soon as you awake and place your feet on the floor.

How many times has this happened to you? You haven't slept much or not at all because of your pain. Upon arising, just moving your body in place, sitting up and putting your feet on the floor causes you to grimace with pain. Every time you do this you are sending out negative vibrations. You're probably not even aware you are doing this because you've done it so many times that it has become a normal routine. Then you take your first step and the first thing that comes out of your mouth or into your thoughts is *$#%! Think about what that is vibrating and you carry that message throughout the rest of your day.

Now is the time to change that habit. As soon as your feet hit the floor and you stand up, clap your hands together three times, throw your hands and arms above your head towards the ceiling, and say out loud (the louder the better) with lots of positive feeling, 'What a 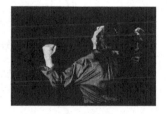 Glorious Day.' Do this two more times (3 times all together).

Even if you don't think it is going to be a glorious day, if you pretend like actors do when playing a character, you will be raising your energy just the same. Your subconscious mind does not know the difference between a lie or a truth. All it knows is the information being fed to it.

Once the information is repeated enough times it becomes its only basis of input and ultimately the information becomes your new truth. When it becomes your new truth, you will vibrate that new truth with a positive emotion that the law of attraction will match.

"We must be willing to get rid of the life we've planned, so as to have the life that is waiting for us. The old skin has to be shed before the new one can come."

Joseph Campbell

Personal Assessment

So you're probably thinking, "I'm pretty sure I already know myself after all these years." Well, that's true for your behavior up to this point. You know yourself by your filters and the stories you've been telling yourself all these years which are called your life scripts.

In childhood you started designing the blueprints of your future life. Within these self-made blueprints you formed who you believe you are by your environment, national history, ethnicity, education, religion, genetics, family, and friends. Most of these inputs are ideas you inherited unknowingly - you simply incorporated then over many years. Some- 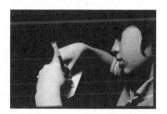 times it could be just a look, a word, a tone, a body language that you emotionally imprinted onto your subconscious mind. Whether they were positive or negative, true or false you kept telling yourself these messages over and over again until they became your truths.

Tony Robbins hit the nail directly on the head when he says, "We are defined by the stories we tell ourselves." The question you should ask yourself is, *are these stories or scripts creating an atmosphere of healing or are they merely keeping you stuck in your pain?*

Think of a time or something that made you feel happy. Why did it make you happy - because it fit your mental picture of the script you created in your mind. So where did this pain you are experiencing right now fit into your blueprint? I guarantee it was never part of it - right? So why are you allowing it to hold you captive? Because you are unaware those old stories are in charge of your current life. If you remain unaware of them then you are at their mercy and you will continually play the victim, never giving yourself the gift of maturity.

Think about those dark nights in your soul, those nights that make you wonder if life is worth living when all you have to look forward to is your pain; those nights when you feel utterly helpless; when you realize your current condition will never change or only get worse. Life looks pretty bleak - right? Well it doesn't have to be.

So how do you start unveiling these life scripts when you're not even aware of them? By your conscious decisions which will become your new destiny.

First, think about the reasons why you are hanging onto your scripts. When you react to a situation or perform a habit, ask yourself if this is true or is this simply your version of reality. Second, ask how is this serving you - are you moving toward or away from your pain?

People tend to live in a black and white world with shades of gray by hanging onto their dis-empowering beliefs. The movie, *Pleasantville*, is a great analogy about living with scripts that no longer serve the people. Humans were created with cones in their eyes to see color with a myriad of hues, tone, contrast, and brightness. That's the way you should be living your life - in full color.

You may not be able to change your present environment but you can change your thoughts that will create a different and better blueprint in spite of your pain.

I'm not saying it will be easy - remember these stories have been who you are throughout your entire life. To be successful in reducing your pain you will have to be vigilant and persistent. Richard St. John sums it up perfectly if you expect any type of success, "you will have to go through CRAP:

> C = criticism
> R = rejection
> A = assholes
> P = pressure"

Changing your life scripts means changing your behavior and that may be uncomfortable for some of the people around you. They are used to the "old" you because your behavior was predictable. When you start changing, it may cause others to question themselves causing them to be uncomfortable with who they believe they are. Be strong for yourself and compassionate for them - remember everything is a process - do you want to remain in pain just to please someone else?

Designing a new blueprint for yourself does not mean you are changing your identity. It means you are expanding it. By taking control of your thoughts, you will:

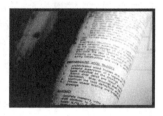

    ...feel better about who you are
    ...have a deeper respect for yourself
    ...be healthier
    ...have better relationships with others
    ...deal with obstacles easier
    ...be in alignment with your values
    ...have clearer paths to achieving your goals

Again, I may sound callus, but I don't care why you are angry, depressed, or frustrated with your pain - your old scripts are driving those messages. I can't change any of your old scripts that are driving those messages. What I care about is helping you change your stories so you can get excited about life again and do all those things you dream about. When you create a new lifescript for yourself, you create a new life that will become more present; and you will no longer be living in the past. By rewriting your stories your attitude will improve - you will no longer be *knee-jerking* to things that come your way.

Let your pain be the element that drives you to a new you - something that causes you to find a deeper meaning to life so you can offer a helping hand to a fellow sufferer. It will fill you on a very deep level because you are totally in control of it.

You are not a leaf in the wind. Life doesn't just happen. You created your life by the stories you've told yourself. You've made choices throughout your entire life controlled by your blueprint. You move toward things that are consistent with your scripts and you move away from things that are not consistent. The choices you make determine your present condition and prepare you for the future. And not doing something or taking an action is a choice as well with consequences.

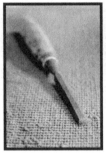

I believe in you - you have the abilities to rewrite your life scripts. Stop letting the "old you" dictate who you are and keep you in pain. Make a new blueprint, chisel a new you. Why would you settle for less? Ask yourself, what are the pay-offs for remaining in pain?

This book is about building layers to start **taming your pain** so take some time to think about your life scripts and how they are serving you right now. Please write down your answers before continuing on.

What are your values and why are they important to you?

What are the negative life scripts attached to your values and how do they hold you back from success? (i.e. I am fat, sloppy, stupid, sick, negative, unfriendly, etc.)

What are the positive life scripts attached to your values and how do they make you feel good about yourself?

What people would be affected by changing your life scripts and how?

A little humor:

HOW DO YOU DECIDE WHO TO MARRY?
(Fun stuff from kids)

1.   HOW DO YOU DECIDE WHO TO MARRY?

You got to find somebody who likes the same stuff. Like, if you like sports, she should like it that you like sports, and she should keep the chips and dip coming.

-- Alan, age 10

No person really decides before they grow up who they're going to marry. God decides it all way before, and you get to find out later who you're stuck with.

-- Kristen, age 10

2. WHAT IS THE RIGHT AGE TO GET
MARRIED ?

Twenty-three is the best age because you know the person FOREVER by then.

-- Camille, age 10

3. HOW CAN A STRANGER TELL IF TWO
PEOPLE ARE MARRIED?

You might have to guess, based on whether they seem to be yelling at the same kids.

-- Derrick, age 8

4. WHAT DO YOU THINK YOUR MUM AND DAD
HAVE IN COMMON?

Both don't want any more kids.

-- Lori, age 8

5. WHAT DO MOST PEOPLE DO ON A DATE?

- Dates are for having fun, and people should use them to get to know each other. Even boys have something to say if you listen long enough.

-- Lynnette, age 8 (isn't she a treasure)

-On the first date, they just tell each other lies and that usually gets them interested enough to go for a second date.

-- Martin, age 10

6. WHEN IS IT OKAY TO KISS SOMEONE?

-When they're rich.

-- Pam , age 7

-The law says you have to be eighteen, so I wouldn't want to mess with that.

- - Curt, age 7

-The rule goes like this: If you kiss someone, then you should marry them and have kids with them. It's the right thing to do.

- - Howard, age 8

7. IS IT BETTER TO BE SINGLE OR MARRIED?

It's better for girls to be single but not for boys. Boys need someone to clean up after them.

-- Anita, age 9   (bless you child)

8. HOW WOULD THE WORLD BE DIFFERENT IF PEOPLE DIDN'T GET MARRIED?

There sure would be a lot of kids to explain, wouldn't there?

-- Kelvin, age 8

9. HOW WOULD YOU MAKE A MARRIAGE WORK?

Tell your wife that she looks pretty, even if she looks like a dump truck. -- Rick, age 7

Raise Your Standards

Ok, now you understand that our behavior is consistent with what we believe we are - our life scripts. So if you believe your life revolves around your pain, that you are unable to do such 'n such because of your pain, then you have become your pain and it now controls you.

I would like you to look backwards and pin-point the time and place where you made that decision. I bet you can't because you have conditioned yourself and adapted a particular behavior pattern regarding your pain over and over again that it has now become your truth. **But it is not the truth and it is not who you truly are.**

You can change your behavioral patterns and beliefs as soon as you make a clear conscious decision to. It's called reprogramming your belief systems. Sometimes it happens in an instant at the time you make an aha or experience a significant emotional event. Other times it happens a bit slower, in fact, so slowly that you may not even notice the shift until you look backwards to see how much has changed.

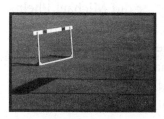 So think about it this way - you are required to raise your standards if you expect to have success in any endeavor you commit to, unless it is failure. There is no such thing as staying in one place. You are either moving in a positive direction or a negative direction.

Your pain, your condition, is a direct reflection of your standards - the identity of your life scripts. So if your identity is being controlled by your pain then your behavior is being controlled by your pain. A wise friend told me once that "behavior never lies". So if your pain is manipulating your behavior then your behavior and your actions determine your results and, in particular, your pain levels. So how are your results working for you so far?

It stands to reason that in order to get better results, you simply raise your standards. Well the concept is a lot easier to say than actually doing the work. You've operated your entire life by your predesignated standards - your life scripts - the stories you've been telling yourself over and over again. You are very comfortable with the stories, in fact you own the stories whether they are working in your best interest or not.

You can change your thoughts in a moment but to have long-lasting results it usually takes a process. Building layer upon layer to create a new standard of behavior, a new habit or way of doing things.

If you want to learn a new skill you must give yourself time to master a new set of behavior patterns by stretching and flexing your muscles both physical and mental. By putting a "carrot" or something rewarding just out of reach, you have something to strive for. You are raising your standards.

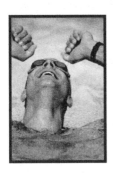 The number one athletes in the world like Venus and Serena Williams did not win their first tennis match on the first or second time they hit a ball over the net. Nor did Michael Phelps take home medal after medal the first time he jumped into a pool. They dedicated their whole lives to being better than anyone else. You bet there were many days they didn't see immediate progress but that didn't deter them. So each time they hit a milestone or won an event, they raised their standards in order to achieve more. They never lost sight of the prize.

So what excites you? What is the catalyst that gets you up in the morning or gives you a reason to live each day? I bet the reasons five or perhaps ten years ago are not the same now that your pain is in control. Right?

So why have you not been able to control your pain up to this point? Perhaps you lack motivation. Motivation means the **act or *process of motivating which is action with an incentive or a force.*** You have been conditioned to believe that no matter what you do, it won't make any difference because, according to your life scripts, your standards have been met.

I want, no I expect, you to raise your standards. It will require a shift in your mindset (life scripts) that you can do because *the rewards are less pain (yeah)*. Raising your standards means having the fortitude to keep going even when you don't see and/ or feel immediate results and a commitment to do your best by fully participating in each activity in this book on a daily basis - believing it will work.

"When you concentrate
your energy purposely on
the future possibility
that you aspire to realize,
your energy is passed on to
it and makes it attracted to
you with a force stronger
than the one you directed
towards it."

Stephen Richards

Law of Attraction

Wikipedia states: "The law of attraction is the name given to the belief that 'like attracts like' and that by focusing on positive or negative thoughts, one can bring about positive or negative results."

In other words, what you focus on or put your attention to will be drawn to you like a magnet. The thoughts and emotions you send out into the universe are what you get more of in return.

A thought creates an emotion. An emotion is a feeling in motion. You don't just feel an emotion, *you do an emotion* which sends out an energy vibration whether it is positive or negative.

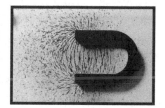

The Law of Attraction cannot discern the difference between positive and negative, good or bad. It responds only to a vibration. It is obedient to what is being put out by a person's thoughts and energy. It can only match positive to positive or negative to negative - nothing more.

According to Michael Losier, an international speaker on the law of attraction, "You may not always get what you want but you will always get what you vibrate."

So if you have become your pain, in other words, your pain is all you think about, feel, and live your life by, that's all you are sending out vibrationally. Therefore, the Law of Attraction is giving more of what you are putting out which is pain and more pain. The universe is always checking and matching - checking what you are vibrating out and matching it.

The good news is that you can change your vibration any time you choose to. The Law of Attraction does not keep score about past events or vibrations, it only matches your current energy output. So with the simple act of choice, you can send out whatever energy you want to manifest back to you.

So how do you do that? By your deliberate choice of thoughts, words, and feelings. You can choose to change your negative basis of judgment (your life scripts) of yourself. If you answered the previous questions honestly, you should start to understand the underlying causes that keep you where you are right now. Just saying positive affirmations is not enough. You have to believe them to be true. It is the positive emotion (remember emotion is a feeling in motion or vibration) behind the affirmation that the universe is matching. Affirmations are a big part of this but not the whole picture. If your words are not in alignment with your feelings, then the law of attraction will only match the feelings.

Did you know that the average person says approximately 300 negative words before noon each day? Now you are not average because you are in the 14 percentile, right, and so the number of negative words for you is less (yeah). Our culture breeds negativity making the number of negative thoughts and words seem normal but if you want to lower your pain levels, you must be aware of certain words like *don't, not and no.*

Don't think of a cat. It is not OK to eat ice cream. No dancing to the music. What did you really think about? A Cheshire or Siamese cat? Vanilla or chocolate ice cream? Dancing to a tango or waltz? Wait a minute, just the oposite of the intension happened. Think about typing the words "not golfing" into a search engine like Google on your computer. Guess what pops up - everything about golfing. This is the similar way the law of attraction works.

If all you know is what you "don't" want then that's all you're going to get more of. *So ask yourself what "do" you want.*

This is a powerful question. Positive things

happen when you start to think and talk in terms of **what you do want** versus what you don't want. Your vibration will change from a negative to a positive and the results of your vibration will be positive. You need to be very clear and specific about what you do want.

Pay attention to how you feel just saying the following sentences:

I don't want a crying baby sitting behind me on the plane.
Vs.
I like quiet and courteous passengers around me when I fly.

I don't want to have to park away from the store entrance.
Vs.
I always find a parking space near the store entrance.

I don't want a lousy job just because I'm not qualified.
Vs.
I am able to learn and be qualified in order to have a good job.

The more you use positive language the more you will recognize the negative language the people around you are using. Instead of affirming their negativity, ask them, *"so what do you want?"* Onc of two things will probably happen: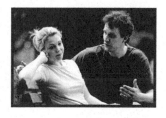
1) The person will stop and think about what you said. At that time you could support them by kindly rewording their complaint into a positive statement.
You will be uplifting the person's energy vibration and he/she will feel good about being around you.
2) People will start avoiding you because you no longer buy into their negative story. They are not interested in raising their energy. Instead they are just looking for someone to feel sorry for them or their circumstances. You will soon discover that long-term associating with this type of people **causes you to lower your own vibration** (is this what you really want to do?).

So when your vibration is high, things come easier for you. You may actually feel lighter. Every time you celebrate the smallest positive event leading to your healing, you raise your vibration.

Practice acknowledging each and every good thing that comes your way. And when you layer one positive on top of another, you are accelerating the effects of the Law of Attraction which brings more good things - more healing equals less pain.

Law of Receiving

The Law of Receiving is the twin of the law of attraction. It does not work for us to go around saying 'I want, I want' even with the highest vibration. You need to make room for the incoming gifts. This is also called the law of reciprocity. When you willingly give, you will graciously receive.

Our bodies are just terminals - a point in which giving and receiving merely change direction. No energy is lost, it is in a constant flow. So in the receiving of a gift, be grateful. The more you give in return the more you will receive.

So many times when we are in pain we find ourselves physically tense and in a blocked state of mind. We literally clench our teeth and are not able to relax. Only when we can relax does the Universe have the opportunity to answer our desires. We have to be open to receiving.

Through a relaxed presence and repetition of gratitude which increases our awareness of life, the more positive gifts flow our way. Everything we are seeking has already been made available. We'll be given it when we have cleared the way for receiving.

It is the thought, the vibration, that attracts the gifts. Billy Graham tells the story about when he and his wife were first married and had no money. At that time $100.00 would just pay for one month's rent and food. On one particular Sunday during the church service as the collection plate was passed to him, he placed in it a one hundred dollar bill and passed it along. After a few minutes he realized what he had done and told his wife that he meant to put in a twenty dollar bill instead of a hundred. His wife looked at him and calmly said, "That's too bad because all the good you're going to receive will only be twenty dollars worth."

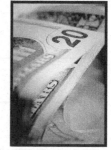

So it is the amount (value) of the thought (vibration) that will be reflected (received) back to you.

Write down some of the negative sentences you say often out loud and to your self.

Now rewrite the negative sentences into positive ones and practice saying them over and over until they become your mantra.

poem

Be Thankful

Be thankful that you don't already have everything
     you desire,
If you did, what would there be to look forward to?

Be thankful when you don't know something
For it gives you the opportunity to learn.

Be thankful for the difficult times.
During those times you grow.

Be thankful for your limitations
Because they give you opportunities for improvement.

Be thankful for each new challenge
Because it will build your strength and character.

Be thankful for your mistakes
They will teach you valuable lessons.

Be thankful when you're tired and weary
Because it means you've made a difference.

It is easy to be thankful for the good things.
A life of rich fulfillment comes to those who are also
     thankful for the setbacks.

GRATITUDE can turn a negative into a positive.
Find a way to be thankful for your troubles and they can
    become your blessings.

~ Author Unknown ~

Gratitude

Gratitude is acknowledging something good has happened or been given to us; a benefit or gift bestowed upon us as we engage our mind in reflection concerning an event. It is also a feeling or emotion that comes from deep inside of us. It percolates from our heart and soul.

Gratitude enriches life and those who express it are happier and enjoy what they have in the present. A person who is happy and thankful lives as much as nine years longer with a better quality of life than someone who is not.

Gratefulness does not depend on wealth, social status, health, or aesthetics. It's a choice we make even in hurtful times. We can choose between forgiveness or bitterness or revenge in any given situation. It doesn't come easily at times as inner growth usually involves some sort of discomfort or pain but in the end, our hearts expand with the grateful lessons learned. Oprah Winfrey says, "We are not what happens to us; we get to choose what to do with what happens to us."

In his book, *thanks! How the new science of gratitude can make you happier,* Robert A. Emmons, Ph.D. and his collaborator, Michael McCullough, set out to prove, or not prove, does being grateful in one's life actually produce happiness. A ten-day experiment was initiated using three groups of people. The first group was asked to write down everything they were grateful for. The second group was asked to write down everything that they were unhappy with in their life. The third group was asked nothing. They found that "participants in the gratitude condition felt more joyful, enthusiastic, interested, attentive, energetic, excited, determined, and strong than those in the hassles condition." It was also noted that their spouses and partners noticed the same affects in the long-term.

On the top of the grateful benefits list was more sleep. Sleep is so vital in restoring the body's ability to repair and heal the wear and tear damages inflicted upon it daily. You can see how this is so true when it comes to pain: pain = less sleep; less sleep = more pain; more pain = less sleep; and even less sleep guarantees more pain. It's a never-ending cycle. Gratitude is one way to help break this slippery slope.

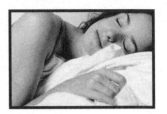

Also, research has shown that when we are grateful, we tend to see more positive things and events around us which are encoded or imprinted into our memory. The deeper the imprinting, the easier and more accessible the past memory becomes. So the more pleasurable our thoughts become the better we feel about ourselves and our environment thus directing our attention away from our pain (remember the law of attraction?).

People who make it a practice to be grateful have shown to increase their wellbeing by 25% over their peers. Since you are already in the 14 percentile of the "normal" population, that number is much higher - you will live longer and happier.

Emmons performed another experiment where he instructed a group of participants to write a 300-word letter of gratitude to someone in their life who deserved thanks but who had not been properly thanked. The assignment was to visit that person and read the letter to them. Not only did the receiver benefit from this display of gratitude, but it is was documented that the author was happier and less depressed afterwards.

The majority of times we associate tears with sadness and/or pain but tears can also be a response to profound gratitude. A positive emotion like deep, sincere gratitude can be overwhelming - it can flood our soul in an instant and open our hearts. Doctors and scientists have recorded and analyzed the heartbeats of people who are unhappy and basically dissatisfied with their life circumstances with those who typically "count their blessings". The unhappy group of people had significantly higher levels of coronary blockage showing more potential for heat attacks.

According to the findings of Rollin McCrafty, Institute of Heart Math, Director of Research, "The heart generates the largest electrmagnetic field in the body. The electrical field as measured by an electrocardiogram (ECG) is about 60 times greater in amplitude than the brain waves recorded in an electroencephalogram (EEG)." After 20 years of research, studies show that positive and/or negative input have a direct affect on our heart beat that can be "detected and measured several feet away from a person's body and between two individuals in close proximity." Wow - even more reason to adopt an attitude of gratitude.

Pain has both physical and emotional affects on our body. Carnigie-Mellon pyschologist Sheldon Cohen found that when a person is filled with gratitude and up-lifting feelings it "provides an inhospitable dwelling place for pain." By seeing your body as a "gift" you bestow a great value to it which means less pain.

Please note that gratitude cannot be bought by another person nor forced upon you by someone giving you a gift. You may have been taught to say thank you out of courtesy but that is just being polite - not genuine gratitude.

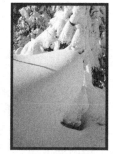

Noting small gratitudes in a journal reminds me of this quote by Daphne Rose Kingman: "Just as millions of snowflakes pile up to create a blanket of snow, the 'thank you's' we say pile up and fall gently upon another until, in our hearts and minds, we are adrift in gratitude."

Being grateful celebrates the good times and events in our lives as well as offering protection in times of pain and crisis. According to Dr. Emmons, "we need to remember the difference between *feeling* grateful and *being* grateful." And David Steindl-Rast, the world's foremost teacher of gratitude has written, "times that challenge us physically, emotionally, and spiritually may make it impossible for us to feel grateful. Yet, we can decide to live gratefully, courageously open to life in all its fullness. By living in the gratefulness we don't feel, we begin to feel the grateful."

The collected studies and evidence of ancient philosophers, theologians, contemporary social sciences, and religious doctrine all state that **having an attitude of gratitude prolongs life and gives meaning to our existence.**

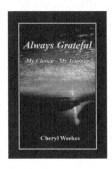

Daily writing in a gratitude journal is the best way to cultivate a grateful heart. You create a record of the blessings which expand upon the sources of goodness. There is no right or wrong way to journal. You could start with a small tablet or a fancy leather-bound book. It doesn't matter. Although I have found that many people, especially if you are new to gratitude journaling, don't know where or how to begin so I have written a book for you called, **Attitude of Gratitude; My Journal, My Choice,** with titles and categories to get you started.

Most people like to write about the pleasantries only but life isn't always pleasant. It's OK to write about the negative (painful) stuff if you found or discovered something to be grateful for "out of the ashes". We all experience days that are so stressful or painful that we simply have nothing good to say. During then, reflecting on better times is helpful like a roof over your head, clothes on your back, food in your stomach, something funny happened in the past, or being able to breathe.

Three things to keep in mind when you start journaling:

... Be aware when you make comparisons. There is always someone physically worse off than you or less educated, or have less money, etc. By making those kinds of "gratitudes" you are actually sending out negative energy instead of positive energy.

... Be conscious about the things and people you may take for granted. Typically we only notice things when they are gone so be mindful of the little things.

... Condition yourself to see the positive in everything. There is never pure good or pure bad, only shades of gray. Our culture tends to exploit the negative so you have the opportunity to counter each time with the positive.

Albert Einstein was not only a brilliant scientist but he had a brilliant grasp on human psychology when he said,

"The greatest thing is to give thanks for everything. He who has learned this knows what it means to live. He has penetrated the whole mystery of life: giving thanks for everything."

"Usually we believe that our pain is a misfortune that needs to be fixed, but in fact, all pain (physical, mental, and emotional) is a necessary step toward becoming conscious."

Eliza Mada Dalian

Acknowledge Your Pain

So you're driving down the road and all of a sudden, for no apparent reason, your car quits running. Turning on your blinker, you coast to the shoulder just before the car stops moving. You get out of the car and walk around it looking for something out of the ordinary to explain the engine failure.

You check the gas gauge - nope, it's OK; then the temperature gauge - nope, it's OK also. You just stand there scratching your head. You try talking to it nicely, "What a nice car you are, I love your paint job, and your interior is still in good shape." When that does nothing to get the car running, you start to shout obscenities at it, "You bla bla bla, who do you think you are leaving me here stranded like this, you are a piece of crap and as soon as we get back I'm trading you in." Nope - that didn't work either.

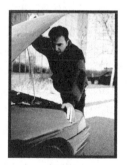

The only thing left to do is to lift up the hood and see what's going on (for the sake of this story you have no cell phone or AAA).Well, this is exactly what you need to do with yourself - you need to look "under the hood" to see what's wrong - what's causing the pain before you can fix it.

For many of us this is stepping into unknown territory. We've hid our pain from ourselves for so long that we are uncomfortable with the idea of facing it. But the only way you can start **taming your pain** and eventually heal is by acknowledging and naming your pain.

Before we can begin to discover the core of our wounds, we need to first address the outward manifestation such as depression, illness, and/or disease. Once we accept and name our symptoms (conditions) we acknowledge that something is "broken" and needs to be fixed in order to move on in our lives. Our pain is simply a sympton of some form of negative energy or imbalance within our bodies.

I bet you are just like me - you have been conditioned to bury your shame, guilt, and hurt throughout your life and move on in order to survive. As a child whenever I complained or behaved poorly I remember my parents telling me to "remember all those starving children in China who have nothing and live in the streets begging for a scrap of food".
Intellectually, I never quite understood what those poor kids in China had to do with me but emotionally, I felt the guilt. The guilt and shame were never addressed so they remained buried in my subconscious mind which became the basis of my life scripts and my pain.

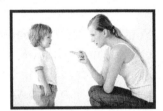

As these "incidences" pile one on top of the other over the years into adulthood, we become numb and/or have the feeling of being emotionally frozen. We ignore our true feelings and start making excuses for our behavior. The buried emotions never go away. Instead they lie in waiting until something happens and our body is in a compromised or weakened state then they show up in illness and disease.

In order to heal any wound, whether physically manifested or emotionally crippling, we need to give it our full attention, or as a certain movie coined the phrase: *the full Monte.*

Pain is pain with different names and causes. The system to bring it to the surface in order to deal with it in a healthy manner will be the same.

Acknowledging your pain is **NOT** a sign of weakness no matter what you've told yourself. In fact, there is no virtue or value in suffering especially when there are techniques to mitigate it. However, it does take courage to accept who you truly are. We are all flawed human beings. The usage of "flawed" in this context means as an imperfection, concealed or not, that impairs soundness and health. No human is exempt from this.

Deborah Kings explains, "Let me be clear: it is not neccessary to vividly recall or relive an event to heal from it. We repress certain experiences because they are too painful or too dangerous. All that is really required for healing is an awareness of how we feel now. If we suspect that our emotions today come from unresolved past experiences, we need to bring the idea of those events into our consciousness without worrying about the details".

How much longer are you willing to carry old burdens and flaws that you built into your life scripts that are keeping you hostage to your pain?

I'm not asking you to look into those dark recesses of your being. Whatever is buried there will percolate to the surface when you are ready and able to address it. Right now we will start with the superficial pain and work backwards to restore health.

So let's open your "hood" and look at the obviously broken item. When that's fixed we can perform more exploration as needed.

Please fill in the blanks in the questionnaire. Be completely honest in order to reap the best benefits for yourself. These answers will be incorporated into the Tapping techniques we will use to start *taming your pain.*

1) What is the name of your pain? _____
   (migraine, sciatica, neuropathy, etc.)

2) Where is it located on your body? _____
   (head, neck, hip, feet, etc.)

3) Describe what the pain feels like? _____

   _____
   (throbbing, hot, cold, numb, etc.)

4) What emotions do you experience? _____

   _____
   (anger, frustration, sad, depression, etc.)

5) Rate your pain level right at this moment: _____
   on a scale of 0 (meaning no pain at all) to 10 (meaning excruciating pain)

Movement Techniques

What I am referring to here is moving the body in gentle gestures. Why is this important to lowering pain levels? Because healing can only occur by moving energy. When we are in pain, we tend to hold our bodies very tightly, tensing our muscles and even shortening our breaths. This in turn, literally blocks the flow of our life-force energy as well as restricts the flow of blood that carries all the elements needed to heal.

When you get a cut on your finger and you put a very tight bandage on it, what happens? The finger starts to turn blue from lack of oxygen and prolongs the healing process. If the bandage is left on long enough, nerve damage may occur and infection. This is the same result with pain and the entire body.

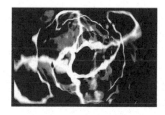 Physicist, Beverly Rubik, discovered that this internal energy, this life-force energy is called 76 different words through the world. The Chinese call it Chi; the Japanese call it Ki; the Polynesians call it Mana, the Hindu call it Prana; etc.

Donna Eden, well known pioneer in energy medicine, believes, "Your body is engineered so that if you tap into the healing force, that force will lead you toward health. It is not just the personality or the soul wanting the body to get better. The *body* wants to heal, and every cell carries extraordinary intelligence and fortitude. While we all sometimes need outside healing and direction, *healing is an inside job*."

This energy force is neither hot nor cold, wet or dry, and is invisible in color. But it can be felt and measured. It runs along channels or pathways called meridians in our body. These are the meridians that acupuncture and acupressure practitioners use in their treatment processes. There are a multitude of reasons that cause these meridians to get sluggish, blocked, and/or even flow backwards depending on the health condition of the individual.

Each meridian is associated with certain organs, muscles, and tissues. When the life-force energy is flowing freely, it produces a positive emotional attribute allowing specific bodily functions to maintain health. But when we experience trauma, either physical or emotional, the energy is impeded causing illness and disease.

So before we can get to the tapping techniques used to address our pain, we need to loosen up the muscles just a bit and get the body in a relaxed mode to allow the energy to start flowing.

The difference between exercise and movement is as follows:

Exercise
- Repetitive movements
- Requires resistance
- Involves pain
- Builds and tones muscles
- Increases stamina
- Good for blood circulations and heart

Movement
- Experience no pain while performing
- Same results with small movements vs large
- Stimulates sluggish/blocked energy pathways
- Opens energy communication to the amygdala
- Improves healing

For the first week, we are going to start off with some very easy, gentle movements.. It is advised that you consult with your physician before doing any of these movements. Do only what is safe and comfortable for you. If you experience any pain as a result of following these suggestions, stop im-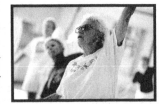

mediately. More pain is not the objective here.

Many people have found that playing healing music in back-groud helps facilitate the healing process. Healing music will be discussed in a later chapter.

Place a sturdy, straight-back chair on a non-skid flooring like carpeting or a yoga mat.

1st Movement

Sit up in the chair with your feet flat on floor – hip
    width apart.
Place two fingers on each of your collar
    bones.
Move your fingers down one inch to indentation between
    the collar bone and top of the first rib.
Gently rub this area in a circular motion as you breathe.
Inhale in through the nose filling the bottom of your lungs.
Hold your breath for 2 seconds.
Exhale out through your mouth.
Repeat the inhale - hold - exhale.

2nd Movement

Place two fingers or your knuckles over the sternum in the
    middle of your chest.
Gently thump your sternum area with a rapid motion as you
    breath.
Inhale in through the nose the filling bottom of your lungs.
Hold your breath for 2 seconds.
Exhale out through your mouth.
Repeat the inhale - hold - exhale.

3rd Movement

Place two fingers about 6 inches below each armpit.
Gently and rapidly thump this area as you breathe.
Inhale in through the nose filling the bottom of your lungs.
Hold your breath for 2 seconds.
Exhale out through your mouth.
Repeat the inhale - hold - exhale.

Slide you fingers under each breast directly below nipples.
Gently and rapidly thump this area while you breathe.
Inhale in through the nose filling the bottom of your lungs.
Hold your breath for 2 seconds.
Exhale out through your mouth.
Repeat the inhale - hold - exhale.

4th Movement

Raise your hands/arms in front of your face.
Place two fingers on the inside of each eyebrow.
Gently massage brows in a circular motion 4 times.
Move your hands over to your ears.
Starting at top of each ear, gentle massage your ears working
    down to the bottom of each lobe.
Repeat this process 3 more times.

5th Movement

Place each pointer finger on the outside corner of each eye.
Place your middle fingers under each eye.
In a circular motion massage all four areas together 4 times.
Reverse direction and massage 4 times.

6th Movement

Place a finger of one hand horizontal under your nose.
Place a finger of other hand horizontal below your lower lip.
At same time massage side to side 4 times.
Drop hands into your lap and breathe.
Inhale in through the nose filling the bottom of your lungs.
Hold your breath for 2 seconds.
Exhale out through your mouth.
Repeat the inhale - hold - exhale.

Now that you have warmed up your meridian areas, you are ready to start tapping.

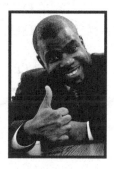

"You need to take responsibility for being the healthiest person you can be. No one else is going to do it for you."

Mehmet Oz, M.D.

Tapping aka EFT

In the early 1970s, David Feinstein, Ph.D. was appointed to the Department of Psychiatry at Johns Hopkins. He was given a special assignment to ascertain if the "new" therapies coming out of the west really worked or were they just California "fluff"? Although he did discover that some of these "new" therapies produced positive changes, he was still holding onto his original tried-and-true beliefs.

Then he was introduced to Energy Psychology; a method using tapping or Emotional Freedom Technique (EFT). In an article he wrote called, *The Case For Energy Psychology*, he states, "I can't fully express how surprised I am to find myself standing here telling you that the key to successful treatment, even with extremely tough cases, can be a mechanical, superficial, ridiculously speedy physical technique that doesn't require a sustained therapeutic relationship, the acquisition of deep insight, or even a serious commitment to personal transformation. Yet, strange as it looks to be tapping on your skin while humming 'Zip-A-Dee-Doo-Dah,' it works!"

Gary Craig was one of those Californians presenting a new way of healing. He took what he learned from Dr. Roger Callahan and organized the techniques so the layperson could easily grasp and perform this new process. He is the founder of Emotional Freedom Technique (EFT) which is now the "Gold Standard for EFT". He offers all of his teachings for free at www.emofree.com.

Since then the Harvard Medical School along with countless case studies and controlled trials using tapping leave no doubt that this method can produce positive outcomes.

A present day pioneer, Nick Ortner who is the CEO of *The Tapping Solution* and Creator and Executive Producer of the breakthrough documentary, *The Tapping Solution* has taken tapping to the public media arena. He has brought together and documented thousands of tapping practitioners' stories along with stories of everyday people just like you and me who experienced physical pain, emotional trauma, phobias, over weight, depression, and/or facing challenges. Each person greatly benefited from using the tapping techniques.

The beautiful thing about tapping is it can be done anywhere, anytime, and you do it to yourself. No special equipment is needed, no pills to take, no doctors needed.

Our body is designed with an amygdala in the mid brain. Scientist have established that this is the *fight-or-flight* response center. Our ancestors required this response mechanism to survive. Without it mankind would have perished but in our present day world we no longer have to fight off dinosaurs or other wild beasts. Yet we still have plenty of stresses - your daughter needs braces, your boss demands more of you than you can handle, the doctor bills are piling up, your car breaks down, the family pet just got ran over, your ailing parents need to move in with you, etc. All of these incidents may not in themselves be overwhelming but add them together and you are in the fight-or-flight mode causing your body to produce significant amounts of cortisol and adrenaline. In short bursts, this protects us from danger but over long periods of time, this causes inflamation, weakens the body's defenses allowing illness and disease to invade.

So how does tapping work? It works on the same principles as acupuncture and acupressure accessing the meridians to "talk" directly to the amygdala. According to Ortner, "What tapping does, with amazing efficiency, is halt the fight-or-fright response and reprogram the brain and body to act - and react - differently."

How? By discharging the negative response we have attached to an event causing us pain. Extensive research using MRI and PET brain scans at Harvard Medical School, have shown the

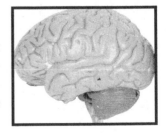

amygdala part of the brain deactivating the alarm components as a result of tapping. In fact, it has proven to suppress the arousal stimuli of the whole limbic system. Also the dehydroepiandros-terone (DHEA) levels in the brain are significantly lowered.

When the arousal of the amygdala is reduced and/or discharged, then the energy trigger of a painful event is no longer activated. Also, the life scripts that we have accepted as our "truth", no longer set off alarms in our brain. The memory remains but there is no nega-tive emotion attached to it.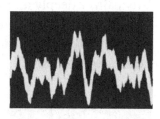

When there is no negative emotion associated to a painful event, the brain is allowed to alter the negative pathways. Because of the neuroplasticity of the brain, these negative pathways are not permanent so you can develop new ways of thinking.

Tapping aligns the body, mind and spirit to feel safe by bringing our attention to the underlying beliefs surrounding the pain in order to reprogram our response.

There are several accupoints throughout our body that connect the meridians to our muscles, tissues and organs. Although en-ergy work includes all of these acupoints, basic tapping uses pri-marily the head and upper body points. Using your fingers to gently tap these points causes an electromagnetic pulse to run along the meridians (a good visual may be fiber-optics in your phone line). For centuries, the Asian cultures have been using these same points to insert, just under the surface of the skin, hair-like needles to produce the same energy pulse.

To begin using tapping may seem a bit awkward. You don't have to do it perfectly just as long as you keep tapping. All of the acu-points send a pulse ultimately to the same place - the amygdala - using different avenues. In the following pages I have named and diagrammed exactly where these points are. Once you do a round or two you will be comfortable with the process.

Since this may be new to you, I have written a very basic script using what is called *the set-up statement*: "Even though I have this pain, I deeply and completely love and accept myself." You cannot lower your pain level and ultimately heal yourself until you verbally acknowledge it. It must be exposed in order to be addressed properly.

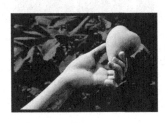 And saying that you love and accept yourself may not be what you truly believe at this moment because of the stories you've been telling yourself all these years. However, remember that your subconscious mind does not know the difference between a lie or the truth, it only knows what it is being told. So by repeating the message that you love and accept yourself, you will be replacing the old message with a new one which in turn will be your new truth. The benefit of choosing to love and accept yourself expands your positive energy field allowing the Law of Attraction to give you what you want - for right now that's less pain.

So, to start a tapping session, you simply begin tapping 6 or 7 times on the points or for as long as it takes to state the phrases. I have outlined in the script for you to say the statements out loud. You'll be filling in the blanks with your own words you previously wrote down on page 56. I have found from personal experience that tapping in front of the mirror augments the process by accessing another part of your brain through sight. The more ways you can get access to your amygdala and subconscious the better the results.

After a tapping session, many people have experienced not only a drop in their pain level but a relaxation in their muscles and their mind is more restful. Aha - the negative energy is dissipating. When your body is relaxed, the healing energy flows unrestricted.

But what if you don't feel better? More than likely it means you need to tap a bit longer. Some people have tapped for very long periods of time before feeling any relief. However, I find that 10 to 20 minutes is sufficient. Then take a break and tap again later throughout the day. It has taken you years to form these patterns of emotional beliefs so be patient and give yourself some time to adjust to a new behavior. Resistance does not mean change can never occur - it will occur with compassion and persistence.

You may find that when you tap about one pain area another one pops up. This is normal. When one area is exposed and the negative energy is discharged, it makes way for other areas to be addressed. We will talk more about this in the next session.

On rare occasions a tapping session may leave you with more pain instead of less. Usually this means there are other very deep-seated emotions that should be addressed by a professional EFT practitioner. Some of the traumas you experienced in your past may be so frightening that you do not feel safe bringing them into your conscious being by yourself. Please do seek help if this happens to you in order to be healthy again.

Typically, tapping brings on a cognitive shift - you become more clear in your thinking because there is less "noise" going on in your head. Noise is that negative chatter that constantly plays over and over in your mind and really serves no purpose other than to bring more stress which reduces our ability to lower our pain. Nick Ortner states, "At the extreme level, this is called the 'Apex Effect'. The Apex Effect happens when a person's thought patterns shift 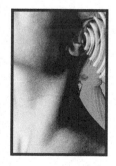 so dramatically that they don't credit tapping as having made a difference. Some even say a belief was never a problem in the first place!"

This is why you write down your pain level before you begin to tap so you have a basis to show progress otherwise you might discount the whole purpose of tapping and not acknowledge its benefits.

Although tapping may seem like a cure to your ailments it is not. By tapping on your past negative emotions, you take away the negative energy associated with a particular event thus making room, freeing you to experience positive emotions and allowing your body to start the self-healing process.

The nine meridian points that we will be using:

Karate Chop points on hands - KC
Head Top center - HT
Inside corner of each Eye Brow - EB
Outer Side corner of each Eye - SE
Under each Eye - UE
Under Nose - UN
Chin Point, under lower lip – CP
Collar Bones - CB
Under Arm pits - UA

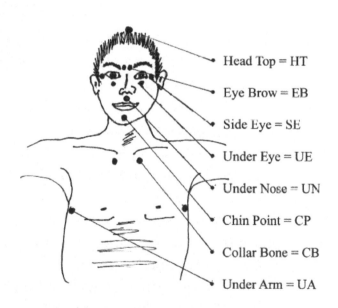

Head Top = HT

Eye Brow = EB

Side Eye = SE

Under Eye = UE

Under Nose = UN

Chin Point = CP

Collar Bone = CB

Under Arm = UA

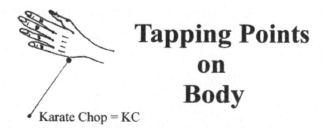

Tapping Points on Body

Karate Chop = KC

Start by filing in the blank areas with the answers you previously wrote down on page 56. Then start tapping on the acupoints
along your body. As you are tapping use the script I have written
for you. We will begin with the set-up statement and add additional words as we go along. This may seem a bit elementary to
repeat these statements so many times but the purpose is to layer
one step at a time in order to change an old pattern of thinking
(one that has kept you in pain) to a new one (one that frees the
negative attachment).

Let's start. You can stand or be seated.....

Round 1:

KC = Even though I have this pain, I
completely and deeply love
and accept myself.

HT = Even though I have this pain, I completely and
deeply love and accept myself.

EB = Even though I have this pain, I completely and
deeply love and accept myself.

SE = Even though I have this pain, I completely and
deeply love and accept myself.

UE = Even though I have this pain, I completely and
deeply love and accept myself.

UN = Even though I have this pain, I completely and
deeply love and accept myself.

CP = Even though I have this pain, I completely and
deeply love and accept myself.

CB = Even though I have this pain, I completely and
deeply love and accept myself.

UA = Even though I have this pain, I completely and
deeply love and accept myself.

Round 2:

KC = Even though I have this _____(name pain from answers), I deeply and completely love and accept myself.

HT = Even though I have this_____(name pain from answers), I deeply and completely love and accept myself.

EB = Even though I have this _____(name pain from answers), I deeply and completely love and accept myself.

SE = Even though I have this _____(name pain from answers), I deeply and completely love and accept myself.

UE = Even though I have this _____(name pain from answers), I deeply and completely love and accept myself.

UN = Even though I have this _____(name pain from answers), I deeply and completely love and accept myself.

CP = Even though I have this _____(name pain from answers), I deeply and completely love and accept myself.

CB = Even though I have this _____(name pain from answers), I deeply and completely love and accept myself.

UA = Even though I have this _____(name pain from answers), I deeply and completely love and accept myself.

Round 3:

KC = Even though I have this _____(name
  pain) in my _____(location), I
  deeply and completely love and accept myself.
HT = Even though I have this _____(name
  pain) in my _____(location), I
  deeply and completely love and accept myself.
EB = Even though I have this _____(name
  pain) in my _____(location), I
  deeply and completely love and accept myself.
SE = Even though I have this _____(name
  pain) in my _____(location), I
  deeply and completely love and accept myself.
UE = Even though I have this _____(name)
  in my _____(location), I
  deeply and completely love and accept myself.
UN = Even though I have this _____ in
  my _____, I deeply and
  completely love and accept myself.
CP = Even though I have this _____ in
  my _____, I deeply and
  completely love and accept myself.
CB = Even though I have this _____ in
  my _____, I deeply and
  completely love and accept myself.
UA = Even though I have this _____in
  my _____, I deeply and
  completely love and accept myself.

Round 4:

KC = Even though I have this _____
         _____(color, name) in my _____ (location),
       I deeply and completely love and accept myself.
HT = Even though I have this _____
         _____(color, name) in my _____ (location),
       I deeply and completely love and accept myself.
EB = Even though I have this _____
         _____(color, name) in my _____ (location),
       I deeply and completely love and accept myself.
SE = Even though I have this _____
         _____(color, name) in my _____ (location),
       I deeply and completely love and accept myself.
UE = Even though I have this _____
         _____(color, name) in my _____ (location),
       I deeply and completely love and accept myself.
UN = Even though I have this _____
         _____(color, name) in my _____ (location),
       I deeply and completely love and accept myself.
CP = Even though I have this _____
         _____(color, name) in my _____ (location),
       I deeply and completely love and accept myself.
CB = Even though I have this _____
         _____(color, name) in my _____ (location),
       I deeply and completely love and accept myself.
UA = Even though I have this _____
         _____(color, name) in my _____ (location),
       I deeply and completely love and accept myself.

Round 5:

HT = This _____
_____(feels like).
EB = This _____(color, name),
SE = in my _____(location).
UE = This _____
_____(feels like)
UN = that makes me so _____
_____(emotion).
CP = I deeply and completely
CB = love and
UA = accept myself.

Round 6:

HT = I'm so tired of having this _____
_____ (feels like)
EB = this _____ (color)
SE = this _____ (name)
UE = that makes me so _____
_____ (emotion)
UN = in my _____ (location)
CP = this _____
_____ (color, feels like)
CB = this _____ (name) that makes me so
_____ (emotion)
UA = this _____
_____ (feels like, color, name).

Round 7:

HT = I am really hurting
EB = Sometimes I feel I can't take anymore
SE = I want to be free of this pain
UE = I've tried so many ways to get well
UN = Nothing seems to work
CP = I'm so exhausted with this pain
CB = I want it to end so I can have my life back
UA = I want to feel calm and relaxed so my body can heal itself

Round 8:

HT = What if I try something new?
EB = I think I may be partly responsible for my pain
SE = I want make healthy choices for myself in order to heal
UE = What would it mean if I chose to be totally responsible for my pain?
UN = I really hate this pain
CP = I'm open to new ways to heal my pain
CB = I choose to treat my body with love and respect
UA = I choose to acknowledge my pain and still love myself

Round 9:

HT = I choose to forgive myself and all those I allowed
      to contribute to my pain
EB = I choose to love myself right here, right now
SE = The more I love myself, the better I take care of
      my body
UE = The more I love myself, I raise my energy level
UN = The more I raise my energy level, the more I'm
      able to love others
CP = I choose to love myself
CB = I choose to release all blockage to my healing
UA = I release those blocks at the cellular level

Round 10:

HT = I love and honor myself at the cellular level
EB = I choose optimum health
SE = I forgive myself for all wrong doings in my life
UE = I choose to forgive the story I have told myself –
      to wipe the slate clean
UN = I choose to be partly responsibility for my pain
CP = What if I choose to take 100% responsibility for
      my healing?
CB = I give my body permission to heal
UA = I deeply and completely love and accept myself

Take 2 deep breaths. Rate your pain level on a scale of
0 (meaning no pain) to 10 (excruciating pain) _____.
Write down your pain level before you tapped _____.
Notice any difference?

Homework for Week 1

Complete the following checklist daily:

Activity	Mon	Tue	Wed	Thur	Fri	Sat	Sun
Glorious Day							
Movements							
Tapping							
Grateful Book							

Write down any insights or "ahas" from this week:

(a little humor)

Wisconsin Farmer

Wisconsin farmer named Ole had a car accident. He was hit by a truck owned by the Eversweet Company, a Harley Westover Company.

In court, the Eversweet Company's hot-shot attorney questioned him thusly:

'Didn't you say to the state trooper at the scene of the accident, 'I'm fine?"

Ole responded: 'vell, I'lla tell you vat happened dere. I'd yust loaded my fav'rit cow, Bessie, into da... '

'I didn't ask for any details', the lawyer interrupted. 'Just answer the question. Did you not say, at the scene of the accident, 'I'm fine!'?'

Ole said, 'vell, I'd yust got Bessie into da trailer and I vas drivin' down da road.... '

The lawyer interrupted again and said, 'Your Honor, I am trying to establish the fact that, at the scene of the accident, this man told the police on the scene that he was fine. Now several weeks after the accident, he is trying to sue my client. I believe he is a fraud. Please tell him to simply answer the question.'

By this time, the Judge was fairly interested in Ole's answer and said to the attorney: 'I'd like to hear what he has to say about his favorite cow, Bessie'.

Ole said: 'Tank you' and proceeded. 'vell as I vas saying, I had yust loaded Bessie, my fav'rit cow, into de trailer and was drivin' her down de road vin dis huge Eversweet truck and trailer came tundering tru a stop sign and hit my trailer right in da side by golly. I was trown into one ditch and Bessie was trown into da udder ditch.

By yimminy yahosaphat I vas hurt, purty durn bad, and didn't want to move. An even vurse dan dat,, I could hear old Bessie a moanin' and a groanin'. I knew she vas in terrible pain yust by her groans.

Shortly after da accident, a policeman on a motorbike showed up. He could hear Bessie a moanin' and a groanin' too, so he vent over to her. After he looked at her, and saw her condition, he took out his gun and shot her right between the eyes.

Den da policeman came across de road, gun still in hand, looked at me, and said, 'How are you feelin'?'

'Now wot da heck vud you say?

"The more you loose
yourself in something
bigger than yourself,
the more energy
you will have."

Norman Vincent Peale

W_{eek} 2
2_{nd} K_{not}

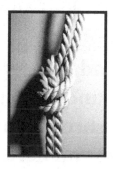

Glorious Day

Since you are in the 14 percentile, I know you have been doing this every morning - congratulations!!! I would like to start out this week sending out positive energy so if it's OK with you, let's do it again before we proceed:

Clap your hands together three times, throw your hands and arms above your head towards the ceiling, and say out loud (the louder the better) **with lots of positive feeling**, 'What a Glorious Day.' Do this two more times (3 times all together).

"I think of all the thousands of billions of steps and missteps and chances and coincidences that have brought me here. Brought you here, and it feels like the biggest miracle in the world."

Lauren Oliver

Littlewood's Law

"Littlewood's Law was framed by Cambridge University Professor John Edensor Littlewood, and published in a 1986 collection of his work, *A Mathematician's Miscellany*. It seeks among other things to debunk one element of supposed supernatural phenomenology and is related to the more general law of truly large numbers, which states that with a sample size large enough, any outrageous thing is likely to happen," according to Wikipedia.

Littlewood used the phrase, one-in-a-million, as a basis for a miracle to happen once in a million exceptional events. He used the assumption that an average person was awake and alert for about 12 hours each day and during that time-frame a person would see or hear one new "event" per second whether it was memorable or not.

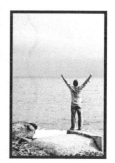

Using this data he concluded that in 35 days, the average person will have experienced about one million events. So by accepting this definition of a miracle, a person could expect to have observed at least one miraculous event during those days.

Therefore, Littlewood concludes that miracles are a common occurrence - one-in-a-million times.

I totally agree and just think of this - you are not average. So does that mean you will have the opportunity to witness even more miracles than the one-in-a million events?

Think about the power of this quote by Albert Einstein and how much it might change your view on life: ***"There are only two ways to live your life. One is as though nothing is a miracle. The other is as though everything is a miracle."***

Evolution has ensured that our brains just aren't equipped to visualize 11 dimensions directly. However, from a purely mathematical point of view it's just as easy to think in 11 dimensions, as it is to think in three or four.

Stephen Hawking

Revolution to Evolution

Revolution means you are ***revving-up to evolve***, to develop and undergo a gradual change. This is what you are doing - you are transforming your life style in order to let your body heal itself as it was designed to.

When you start working on yourself through energy and positive mindfulness, you are able to process information all around you 5 to 10 times greater than your current status. By self-balancing daily occurrences and attending to your health, you will be able to transmute outside influences that could cause more bodily harm.

Unfortunately, many people beat themselves up for being ill for all sorts of reasons. Your life scripts play a big role here as well as perhaps serving other people who are directly involved in your life. Sometimes people are more loving and compassionate to those who are in pain but in the long run, that does not help you get healthy. Neither does judgment or criticism.

Have you noticed that our world is becoming more and more ill? Not just humans but our whole planet. Our "custodians" of earth are polluting our planet and ourselves as humans. It is a mirror affect - we just have to open our eyes to see it.

So the more your thoughts are sending out positive energy, which produces more positive behavior, the more you are able to self-balance to deflect the pollution. When you begin to "wake up" and start getting out of the fog of pain, you will begin to clearly see what's 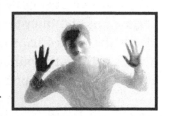 happening all around you that causes pollution to ourselves and the land. Your overall growth (mentally and physically) will slowly produce a positive outcome for all mankind.

The best way to keep people asleep or in a fog is to drug them. As I have previously mentioned, I certainly believe there is a time when drugs are needed with an emergency or to re-balance your emotions or body for a very specific incident. But when a person ingests a drug on a permanent basis, it changes the chemistry 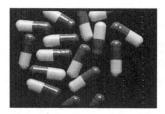 make-up of the body on a cellular level. The body becomes addicted to that drug and/or has a negative reaction which then requires another drug to counteract the initial drug. This causes the body to constantly be a in yo-yo effect allowing for no real healing.

Again, I honestly believe there are people in the drug and medical industry who are ethical and sincere. Sadly, there are those few at the top of organizations who manipulate and intentionally feed the public false information for their own benefit and personal gain. Just like the life scripts you have been telling yourself that you have accepted as truth, these mis-guided individuals have used propaganda to create a certain belief that the public has adopted as truth (remember the subconscious mind only knows what it is told). They spend millions of dollars in advertising and false information to "sell" you an idea and over time you believe what they are selling as your truth.

It is very unfortunate for many people who have suffered dire consequences using/taking certain drugs and have been paid large sums of money to not go public with their story. Fortunately for the rest of us, some of these victims have started telling their stories in the public arena. This awareness is slowly causing a positive change especially in the healthcare industry.

Also, your health is not just determined by the drugs you take but by your environment as well. Daily we are bombarded by negative factors like transportation fumes, microwaves, smog, acid rain, chemicals in our food and water, etc. And we are constantly over stimulated with stress that causes us to end up in the doctor's office where we are given a pill to soothe our aches and pains which only treat the symptons not the causes.

When the drugs don't solve our ailments we turn to alcohol, food, sex, and deviant behavior causing more guilt and damage to ourselves. We get caught up in a slippery slope situation that we have no clue how we got there in the first place or how to get out of it.

Just because you read the articles and see the advertisements doesn't mean you have to believe them as your truth. You are the only one who truly knows your body and what is good and positive for it. Ask yourself for help. Ask your body what it needs to re-balance itself. Ask if your life scripts are true or have they been influenced by the masterful propaganda you see in the media.

Let go of your worry. I know that sounds very simplistic but just start right now. You can't change what has happened in the past or how you have treated your body up to this point but you can accept the fact that the more you educate yourself, the more healthy you will become and thus lower your pain.

Sometimes when we feel quilt and/or remorse we are actually feeling grief for treating ourselves so poorly to allow our health to get to this point. Look at grief as a gift. The gift that you are now waking up and taking positive actions to help your body more than you ever have in the past.

Think of it this way, you can reverse the downhill spiral of deteriorating health: the more you do to lower your pain, the more energy you will have; and the more energy you have, the more you can do to lower your pain. Yeah!

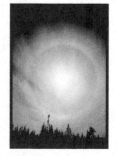

In addition, your body needs a certain amount of sunlight. Just like plants that absorb sunlight to make energy by a process called photosynthesis, your body needs fresh air and sunlight to produce healthy, positive energy. If you spend a lot of time indoors or in darkness you mentally and physically become depressed allowing yourself to be more vulnerable to illness.

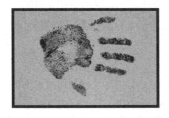 Hold your hand out in front of you with your palm facing you. Look at your palm. You are the only person in the world to have that hand and finger print - that means you are unique - there's nobody created just like you. Your path in life is particular to yourself and you get to choose in what direction and speed you so desire to use. This means your pain and healing is your choice alone.

There is truly nothing outside of you that knows more about you than you. You know what is best for you, you just have to start recognizing your own ability to heal and lower you pain level.

So let's start another revolution to evolution this week. Remember this is a gradual change, one step at a time. What truly matters is that you are here right now in the present. There are three things one must do to be successful in any endeavor:

Show Up
Be Present
Take Action

Congratulations! You are accomplishing all three steps by reading this book and doing the activities. Soooooooooo.........

You will be successful in taming your pain!

My Travels

I have been in many places, but I've never been in Cahoots. Apparently, you can't go alone. You have to be in Cahoots with someone.

I've also never been in Cognito. I hear no one recognizes you there.

I have, however, been in Sane. They don't have an airport; you have to be driven there. I have made several trips there, thanks to my friends, family and work.

I would like to go to Conclusions, but you have to jump, and I'm not too much on physical activity anymore.

I have also been in Doubt. That is a sad place to go, and I try not to visit there too often.

I've been in Flexible, but only when it was very important to stand firm.

Sometimes I'm in Capable, and I go there more often as I'm getting older.

One of my favourite places to be is in Suspense!
It really gets the adrenalin flowing and pumps up the old heart!
At my age I need all the stimuli I can get!

I may have been in Continent, and I don't remember what country I was in. It's an age thing.

"Forgiveness has nothing to do with absolving a criminal of his crime. It has everything to do with relieving oneself of the burdens of being a victim - letting go of the pain and transforming oneself from victim to survivor."

C.R.Strahan

Forgiveness

The word or term *forgiveness* is probably one of the most misunderstood and misused word in any language.

Some people like to throw the word "forgiveness" around like a badge of honor; something that makes them feel like they are a better person than the offender. They feel victimized by the offender so believing if they say they forgive the offense, it makes them the bigger person as if they are offering a gift to the undeserving criminal. In reality, they never truly forgive. They merely seek the feeling of power over the 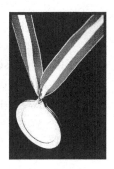 offender by hanging onto the grudge that eventually turns into bitterness. This is another slippery slope that only damages a person by unconsciously augmenting the feeling of a victim, carrying that hurt and pain deep inside them.

According to the book, *Forgiveness: Theory, Research, and Practice,* a biological explanation of an offense is, "The initial damage, or injury to the self, necessarily enters the brain via one of more of the sensorimotor systems. This input is then compared to the existing memory of self and its relationship with the world". (oh, we're back to those life scripts again)

Forgiveness has nothing to do with the offender and everything to do with you. By being wrapped up in the situation, you allow it to remain in power - you find your life being defined by how you were hurt causing you to constantly live in the past. In this state there is no room to live in the present, the now, and no place to move forward with your life; never allowing your body to do what it was designed to do – heal itself. Unconsciously, the buried hurt manifests itself in various physical ailments throughout your body until the offense is forgiven.

Jack Kornfield, in *A Lamp In the Darkness*, states that there are three types of forgiveness:

The first one is forgiveness from others. "There are many ways that [you] have hurt and harmed others, betrayed them, abandoned them, caused them suffering or pain, knowingly or unknowingly," states Kornfield.

The second one is forgiveness for harming ourself. "Just as we have caused suffering to others, there are many ways that we have hurt ourselves. We hurt ourselves at the same time we hurt others. And in many ways we abandon and betray ourselves. The ways you judge yourself about what you've done … and the shame that you still carry in your body, heart, and mind."

The third way is forgiveness of those who have offended us. "Know that [they] have acted this way out of [their] own fear and pain, out of [their] hurt and anger and confusion."

Forgiveness is a choice, a deliberate decision you make for yourself. It is one of the most compassionate acts you can do for your own well being. *You do not deny the pain but acknowledge it and then let it go; a canceling of a debt to yourself or others.*

If you feel you have been harmed by another, it doesn't matter whether the offender accepts or asks for your forgiveness, he/she may never do that so don't expect acknowledgment and/or an apology of any type. As humans we always want to know why; why something bad happened or why someone hurt us so that we may place the appropriate judgment with the appropriate offense. The reason doesn't matter, only our reaction to the situation matters.

There are several methods, techniques, models of behavioral re-enactment and desensitizing practices available through medical professionals but at the very core, the essence, of your belief regarding harm and forgiveness is *your ability to choose your perception.*

Sometimes, forgiveness happens in an instant, other times it takes a while. Forgiveness is a practice. As you discipline yourself to consciously forgive, it becomes a natural part of who you are. It is loving yourself enough to let go of judging and blaming on both sides. It is only through the letting go with compassion, mercy, and tenderness are you able to be set free from the bondage of grievances.

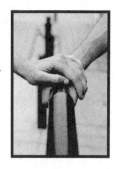

The Law of Attraction states that what you focus on or put your attention to, you draw toward you. If you keep living in the past and constantly blaming or re-dredging the negative events, you are in a perpetual state of agitation (pain). No peace or healing can enter your being. So true forgiveness toward others and yourself allows true forgiveness to be given back to you by all things in the universe.

There are far more benefits to forgiveness than hanging onto grudges and bitterness. Think about it; honest, heart-felt forgiveness means:

a clearer mindset
less anxiety and stress
restful sleeping
being happy
a healthier body
people want to be around you
more fun out of life
spiritually free to receive abundance

Kenneth Pargament sums it up, "forgiveness is a process of re-creation, a transformational method of coping, that involves a basic shift in destinations and pathways in living."

Forgiveness is a choice – a choice only you can make for yourself and no one else.

So if you want to start *taming your pain – start forgiving your pain!*

Forgiveness Assignment:

This week we will be working on the first form of forgiveness which is the harm you have caused others. I chose this one first because, in my opinion, this is the hardest one to forgive.

This requires you to take a long, introspective look into your behavior and how it has affected others around you, personally and professionally.

There are 5 reasons why people hurt others:

> Enjoyment: There is an adrenalin rush of some sort, albeit it is a very negative rush but a rush just the same. There may be the feeling of pleasure because the perpetrator has placed him or her self in a better emotional state than the victim.

> Revenge: One might think that because they have been hurt or wronged that it is OK to do harm back. The media does a great job sending those kinds of messages. Although it makes sensational drama, it teaches the wrong behavior.

> Manipulation: If one does not get a certain expected outcome of an event, many times one justifies using manipulation to eventually turn the issue their way. Again the media is full of stories of characters going behind another's back or spreading false rumors in order to "stack-the-deck" in their favor

> Power: Bullying is a perfect example of abusing one's

position. In the professional arena it might mean belittling an employee in order to boost the ego. Or making fun of a friend or acquaintance in order to be ranked as the "Alfa dog."

Unawareness: We come in contact with people every day that we hardly notice because our minds are so focused on ourselves and what we are going to do when and if bla bla bla. Unaware of how others perceive us may cause them hurt -a certain look or gesture could trigger a negative emotion though no intention was placed on the incident. Also, because we are not mind readers, we may say something innocently but very hurtful to another.

Who are the people you have hurt that you have not made amends with? People who you need to *forgive yourself for any hurt you have caused them.* When you commit your answers to paper, you are bringing awareness to your being so you are able to recognize and address each person in an honest and heart-felt manner.

_____

_____

_____

_____

_____

_____

_____

"Forgiveness is not an occasional act, it is a constant attitude."

Martin Luther King, Jr.

Ho'oponopono & Dr. Hew Len

Ancient Polynesians and Hawaiians called the healing practice of reconciliation and forgiveness ho'oponopono. They believed that all things in the universe are connected (today we call this quantum theory) therefore **all problems originate with thought.**

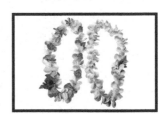

Past events and memories (life scripts) are recorded in our subconscious mind as energy, so in truth, we are 100% responsible for everything and everybody who show up in our life. The average mind receives 11 million bits of data at any given moment. Since the conscious mind cannot analyze that much information at once, it sends 99% of that information to subconscious in order to avoid being overloaded.

Our culture has an addiction to data – we are constantly trying to shove more and more information into ourselves; unaware our egos thrive on it.

Language is data – the story we tell ourselves created in the subconscious - all the negative judgments of being fat, ugly, stupid, etc., along with the positive judgments of smart, healthy, kind, compassionate, etc. Most of these memories whether true or false keep playing over and over again causing the body pain. The subconscious mind cannot discern true or false information – it only receives data. (I don't mean to sound like a broken record by repeating this but it is vital to understand in order to lower your pain levels and eventually heal).

God, Source, Divine, Universe did not create people to continually be in pain so why do we have it? Pain is the negative energy stored in the body. It is telling us to "stop" doing whatever we keep doing to ourselves. Pain is the result of "stuff" within us, not outside of us. Pain is the language, the data, the story we keep replaying in our subconscious mind. We choose to be in pain by our story. Lingering or chronic health problems are not caused by another person or virus or accident – they are caused by what we choose to hang onto; the story we told ourselves a long time ago. Chronic pain is the memory of a past event buried in our subconscious mind that we are emotionally reacting to whether we are aware of it or not. *(back to those life scripts again)*

 We are 100% responsible for everything and everyone that shows up in our life because everything and everybody are connected in this universe. Ho'oponopono is the way to erase the past - to clean the slate containing old data and memories that no longer serve us. It creates a state of blank/void (quantum physics calls this the phantom portal). Ho'oponopono removes all the negative energy so our body can do what it wants to do - heal. This clearing or voiding allows freedom so inspiration can come into your being.

Dr. Ihaleakala Hew Len, renowned ho'oponopono specialist, says, "My job here on earth is twofold. My job is first of all to make amends. My second job is to awaken people who might be asleep. Almost everyone is asleep! The only way I can awaken them is to work on myself."

For 3 years Dr. Hew Len worked at the Hawaii State Hospital for the criminally insane. He never once encountered any of the patients in the hospital. Instead he sat in an office by himself and just reviewed individual files. Each day he would work on himself so whenever a thought or feeling came to him, he would turn it over to the Divine with ho'oponopono because he knew that each individual's actions were showing him a part of himself that needed to be healed.

Over time the patients began to heal themselves and were eventually released. In 1987, the hospital was emptied of patients and closed, never to be opened again.

So how did Dr. Hew Lin accomplish such a feat and what does he believe?

Dr. Hew Len believes our mind's view of our world is through very limited filters that are incomplete and/or inaccurate and we must clean and clear everything in order to be healthy.

A person cannot purify him or her self, only the energy associated with that person. You don't have to know what the past problems are – all you have to do is notice them.

Our present day environment keeps us in a constant state of anxiety and turmoil. We must perform a clearing to remove all negative energy - remove all thinking or nonthinking thoughts to heal and stay healthy. If you have a negative encounter with someone, it is not with that other person but with yourself. The same applies to a health issue - it is the memory of a passed event buried in your subconscious mind that you are reacting to. Whatever shows up in your life *is about your life* even if you are not consciously aware of it.

When you clear your mind to zero, void of data, inspiration comes in. Inspiration (in-spirit) is God, the Divine, Universe, where everything is available – including healing.

How do you do ho'oponopono?
By saying this prayer to your Creator:

I'm Sorry
Please Forgive Me
Thank You
I Love You

What does *"I'm Sorry"* mean?

Sorry for the past energy, actions, and/or deeds that you have caused which brought pain to yourself and others. You don't have to know the how, when, or where of the violation. There is no right or wrong – no judgment involving any and all events you brought into your life because everything is connected. You just have to take 100 % responsibility and you must be completely sincere.

What does *"Please Forgive Me"* mean?

You are repenting for all the past events, known or unknown. You are asking for forgiveness of your actions and those of others in your life without blame or judgment; clearing the slate of all wrong doing; and neutralizing all emotions of anger, fear, resentment, mistrust, blame, etc. Through forgiveness, you are creating a new slate of emptiness, void and/or nothing, and removing the past connection to data.

What does *"Thank You"* mean?

Thanking God for the opportunity to clear the slate of all negative energy. Being grateful for a new, fresh start - setting yourself free from the bondage, chaos, and past perceptions of the subconscious mind.

What does *"I Love You"* mean?

You are connecting back to Source by letting pure love flow into your being and experiencing all that the Divine has to offer you. With the energy of love, you are open for God to fill you with goodness and abundance.

Do-A-Dare-A-Day

Now we are going to jump from the emotional to the physical. Over the years you probably have become quite comfortable with your daily routines and lifestyle. Well, this is where I want you to start stepping out of your comfort zone.

Scientist have measured the retention/memory of listeners and readers after 4 weeks time and found that only 10% of the information received was retrievable. When the subjects took notes, they could remember about 50% of the same information. Only when the subjects were emotionally and physically involved were they able to remember 90% to 95% of the materials presented. Being physical and tapping into the emotions drives the message into several places in the brain.

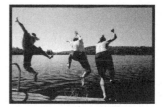

In order to become more than you are right now, to grow and change your behavior patterns, you need to do something different from what you always do.

Concider all the little things you do without thinking about the mechanics of the action. The majority of the time you move throughout your day in rote. I want you to be more aware and not take so many things for granted.

Do-A-Dare-A-Day is doing something different. You can start off with something simple like brushing your teeth. If you are right-handed, switch hands - use your left hand throughout the whole process. If you eat using your left hand to hold the utensil, eat with the opposite hand. Drive a different route to work. Walk backwards down the hallway.

Don't be afraid to do something new. This may be difficult at first try but don't give up and quit - keep going. You are the right person in the right place at the right time to experience this endeavor.

Each day I want you to do one thing outside of your normal routine.

What is your dare? _____

_____

How many times did you do it? _____

How did it feel? _____

_____

What were the ahas you gained from this endeavor? _____

_____

_____

_____

_____

Balance & Your Pain

As we have discussed previously, when we are experiencing pain, we tend to hold our body tightly. The pain reduces us mentally, makes us feel small emotionally, and because we are not able to stand tall, it reduces us physically as well.

Because we are not able to stand erect as we were designed to do, our balance becomes challenged. Our balance is not only regulated by the inner ears, muscles and tendons in our feet, it is also determined by our posture. So when our body is compromised by our pain, it compensates the best way it can.

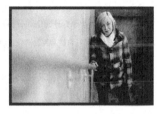

Also, pain can damage the nerves at the neuromuscular junction where the motor neurons meet the muscular fibers, stimulating contractions necessary for movement. This causes shifts in the foot positioning which may change your center of gravity. It also may cause changes in your gait; normally walking heel to toes may cause enough pain that you start walking on the sides of your feet causing awkward balance and instability.

The body's ability to sense movement within joints and joint position is called proprioception. This ability enables us to know where our feet and hands are without having to look at them directly. It is important in all of our everyday movement. Receptor nerves are positioned in the muscles, joints and ligaments around joints and in a healthy system, can sense tension, pass this information to the brain where it is processed, and then send it back to the muscles to contract or relax in order to produce the desired movement. This whole system is subconscious. We don't consciously have to think about the process – it is reflexive. But with chronic pain these receptors can be damaged causing a delay or no response at all.

Our muscles, joints, and tendons become rigid and inflexible without proper movement. "Balance exercises are specific activities that help build lower extremity (or leg) muscle strength as well as improve your vestibular system, the organ associated with balance perception. Balance exercises are particularly beneficial ...as they have been shown to help prevent falls. Each year, U.S. hospitals have 300,000 admissions for broken hips, and falling is often the cause of those fractures. Balance exercises can help you stay independent by helping avoid disabilities that may result from falling," to quote Laura Inverarity, D.O. in the article, *An Overview of Balance Exercises*, for www.about.com.

Exercise can be greatly beneficial in mending damaged sensory nerves. It strengthens weak muscles due to lack of use, helps with range of motion, improves balance and circulation, and reduces swelling of the extremities.

So by doing the following exercises, you will be accomplishing four things:
> 1) increasing the blood flow to the damage nerves for healing
> 2) increasing the functioning of the mitochondria (energy) in the cells
> 3) allowing the body to more efficiently utilize nutrients
> 4) increasing endorphins which makes us feel good and reduces pain

Before you start any exercise regime, you should consult with your physician. Only do as much or as little that you are comfortable doing. You are in enough pain right now that you don't need to add to it.

It is best to find a partner who can help with these exercises by timing you and standing close in case you fall. If that's not possible, count the seconds yourself.

You will need a very sturdy chair that you can hang onto. It's best to do these simple steps ***barefoot*** on a hard, flat surface.

Stand and face the back of the chair. Hold onto the back with both hands for balance. If you feel safe to hold on with one hand, turn sideways to the back of the chair.

Round One:

With both feet flat on the floor, raise your toes up off the floor then lower them back to the floor. Now raise your heels off the floor and back down to the floor. Repeat this process 5 times.

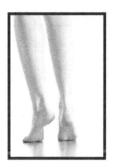

With both feet flat on the floor, roll the sides of your feet in, toward each other and then back. Now roll the sides of your feet to the outside of feet and then back. Repeat this process 5 times.

Round Two:

Lift one foot off the floor while bending the same knee about a 45 degree angle. Start counting (one-one thousand, two-one thousand, etc.) to see how long you are able to balance in this position before you have to put your foot down to regain your balance.

Write down the number in the Balance Worksheet – Eyes Open space on the next page. Repeat the same process two more times. Then total the numbers and divide by 3 to get the average number. Fill in the spaces provided.

Now repeat the exercise using the other leg and fill in the numbers.

This time, close your eyes and perform the same tasks as above. Fill in the numbers on the Balance Worksheet – Eyes Closed on the next pages.

Balance Time Sheet - Eyes Open

Date	1st Set	2nd Set	3rd Set	Total	Average

Balance Time Sheet - Eyes Closed

Date	1st Set	2nd Set	3rd Set	Total	Average

What's Your Balance-Based Real Age?

Compare your numbers with the balance-based RealAge chart below.

Do not be discouraged by your numbers. By doing these exercises once or twice a day, you will be able to track your improvement and strengthen your muscles in order to prevent possible falls and/or injuries.

Balance Time	Balance Age
4 seconds	70 years
5 seconds	65 years
7 seconds	60 years
8 seconds	55 years
9 seconds	50 years
12 seconds	45 years
16 seconds	40 years
22 seconds	30-35 years
28 seconds	25-30 years

www..RealAge.com Copyright © 2013, RealAge, Inc.

I was shocked the first time I did the balance exercises and discovered the results but in time, I was able to match and even improve on the holding seconds. *So can you!*

More Movements

Each week we will be adding a few more movements tucked onto the preceding ones. As you become more comfortable with change, it will be easier to adapt to more and more new concepts and activities. The following new movements are designed to allow your body to become more flexible and less congested.

We will start with week 1's program (go to page 59) and then continue with these new movements:

7th Movement:

Still sitting in the chair, place your hands on your knees and
      lean forward.
Roll your shoulders and body in a circular motion working up,
      to one side, then down, and up to the other side.
Make 4 complete circles.
Reverse direction and make 4 more complete circles.
Come back up to an upright sitting position.

8th Movement:

Drop down forward and lean your elbows on top of your knees.
Shift your weight and move your body side to side 4 times.
Come back up to a sitting position.
Inhale in through the nose filling the bottom of your lungs.
Hold your breath for 2 seconds.
Exhale out through your mouth.
Repeat the inhale - hold - exhale.

9th Movement:

Grab both sides of chair seat with each hand.
Move your body side to side 4 times.
Lean your body to the left and place your right hand over chest.
Raise your right elbow to shoulder height.
Breathing in, reach your elbow across your body
Breathing out, return your elbow/arm back to the side of your
        body.
Repeat 3 more times.
Drop your hand and grab side of chair.
Lean your body to the right and place your left hand over chest.
Raise your left elbow to shoulder height.
Breathing in, reach your elbow across your body.
Breathing out, return your elbow/arm back to the side of your
        body
Repeat 3 more times.
Drop your hands into your lap and come up to a sitting position.
Inhale in through the nose filling the bottom of your lungs.
Hold your breath for 2 seconds.
Exhale out through your mouth.
Repeat the inhale - hold - exhale.

Now you are ready to start another tapping session.

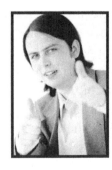

Tapping Plus More

How's the tapping been going so far? Have you noticed any new things pop up - like pain in other parts of your body or things or people you haven't thought about for ages? Since tapping is connecting with your subconscious mind you may find thoughts that were buried and long since forgotten start to surface. This is a normal process of your subconscious doing some house cleaning.

Write down any new thoughts that have surfaced throughout the week even if they seem silly or insignificant. We will be reviewing them later for future tapping sessions.

_____

_____

_____

_____

_____

_____

_____

_____

_____

_____

Just as with adding a few new movements to your routine, we are adding a few new tapping statements. Only you don't have to repeat last week's statements - you will start tapping with the following new script. Before we begin, rate your pain level from 0 (meaning no pain) to 10 (meaning excruciating pain) _____.

Round 1: (see page 69 for chart)

HT = I really hate this pain
EB = I am really hurting
SE = I feel there is so little I can do to stop it
UE = I wish it would just end
UN = This _____(feels like)
CP = This _____ (color)
                _____ (name)
CP = In my _____ (location)
CB = There seems to be no relief
UR = I'm so frustrated with this constant pain

Round 2:

HT = This pain is causing so much stress
EB = I don't know how much longer I can take it
SE = I've tried so many methods
UE = So many different techniques
UN = And nothing has worked so far
CP = I want this pain to stop
CB = I blame myself
UA = How could I have let this pain control me

Round 3:

HT = Even though I still have this pain
EB = This _____ (name)
SE = In my _____ (location)
UE = This _____ (color) pain
UN = This _____ (feels like)
CP = That makes me feel so _____
_____ (emotion)
CB = I deeply and completely
UA = Love and accept myself

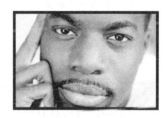

Round 4:

HT = I'm tired of blaming myself
EB = I'm tired of blaming others
SE = It makes no difference
UE = I still have this awful pain
UN = This pain that controls my life
CP = That keeps me frustrated and angry
CB = This pain that is keeping me a prisoner
UA = I want to be free of it

Round 5:

HT = Even though I doubt it will ever go away
EB = I want to rest and be calm
SE = I need to rest and be calm
UE = I want to do something to stop it
UN = I'm open to new ways of healing
CP = I accept new possibilities of being pain free
CB = I really would like to feel better
UA = I want to be happy again

Round 6:

HT = I've forgotten what it feels like to be healthy
EB = I'm in so much pain
SE = This awful _____ (name)
UE = _____ (color)
UN = This _____(feels like)
CP = I'm so tired of this pain
CB = And it's wearing me down
UA = I want to rest and be calm

Round 7:

HT = Even though I have this pain
EB = I really do love myself
SE = I really do accept myself just as I am right now
UE = I release all this pain
UN = I release it at the cellular level
CP = I no longer desire to be in pain
CB = To let this pain run my life
UA = I completely and deeply love myself.

Take two deep breaths and relax. What is your pain level right now? _____

The Road Not Taken

by
Robert Frost

TWO roads diverged in a yellow wood,
And sorry I could not travel both
And be one traveler, long I stood
And looked down one as far as I could
To where it bent in the undergrowth;

Then took the other, as just as fair,
And having perhaps the better claim,
Because it was grassy and wanted wear;
Though as for that the passing there
Had worn them really about the same,

And both that morning equally lay
In leaves no step had trodden black.
Oh, I kept the first for another day!
Yet knowing how way leads on to way,
I doubted if I should ever come back.

I shall be telling this with a sigh
Somewhere ages and ages hence:
Two roads diverged in a wood, and I—
I took the one less traveled by,
And that has made all the difference.

Start Living a Positive Life

The majority of people who are in chronic pain become very myopic in their view of the world around them. They think only of themselves and their pain. Of course that is NOT you because you are that one in seven people who really want to relieve your pain and start living a normal, healthy life again. That includes being productive as well - stepping out of your cocoon, this web of pain that has enveloped you.

Living a positive lifestyle is a choice. In fact, *all of life is a choice.* So many of us have been shut down for so long that we don't know where or how to start living again. Think back to a time when your pain did not restrain your activities. What made you happy? What gave meaning to you? What inspired you to do more? What and who made you laugh?

There are so many things you can do starting right now, in spite of your pain. Remember you are responsible for taming your pain and only you. Everything you have done so far has brought you to this point. When you get yourself out of the way, life becomes more enjoyable; when you are enjoying yourself, you experience less pain; when your experience less pain, your body can heal itself.

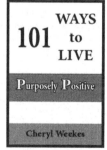

If you are having difficulties thinking of something positive that you could do starting today, read my book, *101 Ways to Live Purposely Positive*, for suggestions.

Happiness is a choice and so is your unhappiness. *Start finding joy by giving of yourself to a cause other than your pain.* Happiness is derived by directing energy and seeing progress in a positive outcome. Yes, it may be scary to step out since it's been so long but trust me, when you do that's when true healing begins. Bringing joy and light into your life is the most loving thing you can do for yourself and others.

Write down 3 things you might like to do to start living again:

1) _____

2) _____

3) _____

Now pick one to start with. Make a commitment to do it today-there may never be a tomorrow. Write out the steps you need to take, the people you need to contact, and the time-frame that is needed to accomplish the task. Mark it on your calendar and make it a priority. *This is a life-changing experience!* So far what you have been doing to expose yourself to life has not been helpful. Give yourself permission to get back into life and start .... *taming your pain. You can do this!*

My first positive lifestyle is _____

In order to do this, I need to arrange _____

_____

_____

The date and time I am able to do this is _____

_____

By signing this, I am fully committed to see this positive action through to completion:

_____

Homework for Week 2

Complete the following checklist daily:

Activity	Mon	Tue	Wed	Thur	Fri	Sat	Sun
Glorious Day							
Forgivenss							
Hoʻopono-pono							
Do-a-Dare-a-Day							
Balance Exercises							
Movements							
Tapping							
Positive Action							
Grateful Book							

Write down any insights or ahas from this week:

_____

_____

_____

_____

_____

_____

_____

_____

_____

_____

_____

humor:

Who's Driving Whom?

After getting all of Pope Benedict's luggage loaded into the limo, (and he doesn't travel light), the driver notices the Pope is still standing on the curb.

"Excuse me, Your Holiness," says the driver, "Would you please take your seat so we can leave?"

"Well, to tell you the truth," says the Pope, "they never let me drive at the Vatican when I was a cardinal, and I'd really like to drive today."

"I'm sorry, Your Holiness, but I cannot let you do that. I'd lose my job! What if something should happen," protests the driver, wishing he'd never gone to work that morning.

"Who's going to tell," says the Pope with a smile.

Reluctantly, the driver gets in the back as the Pope climbs in behind the wheel. The driver quickly regrets his decision when, after exiting the airport, the Pontiff floors it, accelerating the limo to 205 kms. (about 127 mph)

"Please slow down, Your Holiness," pleads the worried driver, but the Pope keeps the pedal to the metal until they hear sirens.

"Oh, dear God, I'm going to lose my license -- and my job," moans the driver as he notices a police car chasing them.

The Pope pulls over and rolls down the window as the cop approaches, but the cop takes one look at him, goes back to his motorcycle, and gets on the radio.

"I need to talk to the Chief," he says to the dispatcher.

The Chief gets on the radio and the cop tells him that he's stopped a limo going 205 kph. "So bust him," says the Chief.

"I don't think we want to do that, he's really important," said the cop.

The Chief exclaimed, "All the more reason!"

"No, I mean really important," said the cop with a bit of persistence..

The Chief then asked, "Who do you have there, the mayor?"

Cop: "Bigger."

Chief: "A senator?"

Cop: "Bigger."

Chief: "The Prime Minister?"

Cop: "Bigger."

"Well," said the Chief, "who is it?"

Cop: "I think it's God!"

The Chief is even more puzzled and curious, "What makes you think it's God?"

Cop: "His chauffeur is the Pope!"

W_{eek} 3

3_{rd} K_{not}

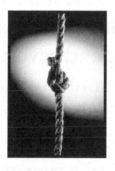

Glorious Day

Congratulations - you've made it to week three!!!

As before, I would like to start out this week sending out positive energy so if it's OK with you, let's do it again before we proceed:

Clap your hands together three times, throw your hands and arms above your head towards the ceiling, and say out loud (the louder the better) **with lots of positive feeling**, 'What a Glorious Day.' Do this two more times (3 times all together).

"While it is true that many people simply can't afford to pay more for food, either in money or time or both, many more of us can. After all, just in the last decade or two we've somehow found the time in the day to spend several hours on the internet and the money in the budget not only to pay for broadband service, but to cover a second phone bill and a new monthly bill for television, formerly free. For the majority of Americans, spending more for better food is less a matter of ability than priority."

Michael Pollan

Nutrition

Well, I bet you think this chapter is going to tell you about a newly discovered plant that grows in the jungle and all you have to do is incorporate it into this fabulous diet that is guaranteed to make the pain go away - right?   Wrong!

You've heard the old saying: you are what you eat. What I am going to talk about will open your eyes to a whole new way of looking at what you put into your body and how it is keeping you in pain. And if you continue to eat the foods you do, you will only become more and more toxic and ill.

I'm talking about Genetically Modified Organism (GMO) or Genetically Engineered (GM) foods. These are foods that scientists are playing "God" with. They have removed a portion of a gene on one organism and replaced it with a portion of a gene from another organism to recreate a new, unknown in nature, organism. The reason for this is to produce crops that are RoundUp resistant and insect resistant.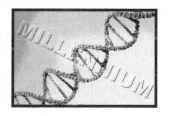

The Food and Drug Administration (FDA) has been lying to the public since 1992 when this new technology started to be used in mass production.

In 1999, scientists and doctors had proof that the GMO foods were dangerous to consume by humans and animals when an epidemic called eosinophilia myalgia syndrome (EMS) broke out. L-tryptophan made by Showa Denko imported from Japan was the only link between over 10,000 people who got sick, some permanently disabled, and 100 people dead. To make the product more economical and produce high concentrations of several enzymes, genes had been inserted into bacteria's DNA causing a mutation that proved to be disasterous.

That's just one case. Since the introduction of GMOs, there has been an increase in: Inflammatory Bowel Disease, Ulcerated Colitis, chronic constipation, gastrointestinal infections, Crohn's Disease, gastrointestinal reflux, allergies, auto immune disease, heart disease, kidney and liver disease, diabetes, and many more.

Why? Because t*he signature of a GMO gene does not exist in nature, it's a man-made creation.* So our body, and those of animals, looks at this "new" gene and views it as a foreigner, an enemy, and attacks it. When this happens, inflammation occurs and long-term inflammation leads to illness and disease.

When anyone in the scientific community has spoken out publically against the use of GMOs, they "have been attacked, gagged, fired, threatened, and denied funding....Attempts by media to expose problems are also often censored," according to the Institute For Responsible Technology. The remaining majority who find problems with GMOs are now employed by the same companies who produce GMOs. This is also happening with former and current persons in charge of policy within the FDA.

Thankfully the American Academy of Environmental Medicine took a very strong position against GMOs because, "animal studies indicated serious health risks associated with GMO consumption including infertility, immune dysregulation, accelerated aging, dysregulation of genes associated with cholesterol synthetics, insulin regulation, cell signature, and protein formation, and changes in the liver, kidney, spleen and gastrointestinal systems."

GMOs have been banned in France, Luxembourg, Germany, Austria, Hungry, and Greece for human consumption. The sad part is that GMOs are being imported (primarily from South America) to these countries as livestock feed which filters back into the human body when these animals are eaten.

Mexico has also banned GMOs but receives nearly 40% of its industrial corn (GMO) from the US to feed livestock.

GMO crops cover 250 million acres worldwide and 80% of the industrial crops grown in the US are GMOs. Next time you go to the grocery store, think about this; 70% of what is on the shelves are GMO foods.

So what is the purpose for GMOs? By modifying the genes of certain plants, these "new"plants will not die when the fields are sprayed with a herbicide to kill off the other vegetation. Basically the herbicide deprives the other vegetation's ability to absorb nutrients so by weakening the vegetation's defense mechanisms, it cannot fight off diseases and bacterium from the soil and dies. So when humans 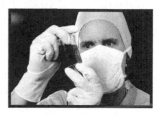 and animals ingest GMO foods, we become deprived of nutrients as well, primarily copper, zinc and magnesium.

RoundUp is the number one herbicide (weed killer) used today throughout the world. Glyphosate is the main ingredient in RoundUp. According to an article in Natures Country Store, "A recent study by eminent oncologists Dr. Lennart Hardell and Dr. Mikail Eriskson of Sweden, has revealed clear links between one of the world's biggest selling herbicide, glyphosate, to non-Hodgkin's lymphoma, a form of cancer."

In a report put out by the Environmental Protection Agency and the World Health Organization, glyphosate affects the adrenals causing insomnia and was found to cause significant DNA damage to the erythrocytes (red blood cells) causing hypoxia, difficulties in breathing, chest pains, and confusion.

The article from Natures Country Store goes on to say, "RoundUp causes damage to the liver that inhibits the liver's ability to process toxic substances...Testing of patients suffering RoundUp exposure has indicated damage to their P-450 enzyme system... The P-450 enzyme system is one of the main body systems for detoxifying harmful chemicals. When it becomes impaired by those same chemicals it is supposed to be detoxifying, the effects of a given chemical on the body increase dramatically." Studies have shown that taking Tagamet, Axid, Pepsid, and/or other H-2 Blockers (antacids) reduce the body's ability to detoxify Round-Up.

"Until now, most health studies have focused on the safety of glyphosate, rather than the mixture of ingredients found in Roundup. But in the new study, scientists found that Roundup's inert ingredients amplified the toxic effect on human cells—even at concentrations much more diluted than those used on farms and lawns", wrote Crystal Gammon in article called *Weed-Whacking Herbicide Proves Deadly to Human Cells* for Scientific American magazine.

Gammon goes on to say, "One specific inert ingredient, polyethoxylated tallowamine, or POEA, was more deadly to human embryonic, placental and umbilical cord cells than the herbicide itself – a finding the researchers call 'astonishing.'"

POEA is a surfactant that breaks down the plant's natural ability to shed liquids allowing the toxic ingredients to penetrate the plant's inner living system. POEA acts the same way detergents do to break down grease molecules on dirty dishes.

This seemingly "inert" ingredient helps increase the toxicity of RoundUp's main ingredient by penetrating clothing, equipment, and the human cells.

So who developed glyphosate, the main ingredient in Round-Up? Monsanto - that is John E. Franz, an organic chemist, while working his entire career at the Monsanto Company in 1970. It only took four years before it hit the market under the name of RoundUp.

During the Viet Nam War, Monsanto along with Dow Chemical produced *Lasso* herbicide, aka *Agent Orange*, used as a defoliant resulting in over 400,000 deaths and disabilities (including our own veterans) and over 500,000 children born with disabilities.

Monsanto was accused of manipulating and falsifying data given to the FDA resulting in thousands of veteran's denial of benefits. Even though there were requests made to investigate the findings, none were made. In 1984, Monsanto was named as one of the seven companies that paid out $180 million to settle out of court and a little over 45% of that amount was paid by Monsanto. This topic is still being fought in the courts today.

When the war was over, there was no more market for Lasso so Monsanto devoted the majority of its efforts to GMOs. Between 1995 and 2005, Monsanto had incorporated over 50 seed companies world-wide threatening the extinction of natural food crops in the very near future.

So in the US alone 80% of the crops are GMO food - corn being the number one product. Soy is number two - also known as Soya, mono-triglyceride, Soja, Yuba, TSF (textured soy flour), TSP (textured soy protein), TVP (textured vegetable protein), lecithin, and 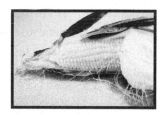 MSG. Genetically engineered soy behaves a bit different than corn - it mimics estrogen causing gynecoastic (breast enlargement), mood swings, crying spells, erectile dysfunction, and lower sperm count in men. In women, GMO soy has been known to increase risks for developing retrograde menstruation where the menstrual cycle backs up into the body instead of flowing out. This can cause endometriosis and eventually cause infertility.

Currently Monsanto produces over 20 GMO crops and it about to introduce a GMO apple called, Arctic Apple.

In 2006, Monsanto filed patents on intellectual properties making farmers sign agreements to "respect the company's patent on the modified gene", meaning that farmers are forbidden to save GMO seeds to replant the next year. Monsanto has become so powerful that they have their own "gene police" who investigate farmers on a regular basis to insure no GMO seeds are on the premises unless authorized (at a fee) by Monsanto.

Many farmers rightfully or wrongfully accused are either forced to sell their land and/or are bankrupted. A phone number of 1-800-roundup is given to all farmers using GMO crops/seeds to snitch on their neighbors for a reward.

This is how powerful this company has become. Many high-ranking people in the US government have either previously worked for Monsanto or left their government positions to work for Monsanto, either way they are highly influenced. During the Bush administration, Monsanto was given the right to not have to answer to the EPA for regulations and the FDA has ignored requests for investigations into scientific studies, performed outside of Monsanto's laboratories, of the effects of GMOs. Although Monsanto claims that GMOs are safe, there has been no long-term data provided so far by the company.

OK, sorry that I got side-tracked there but I thought it was important to help put things into perspective. However, RoundUp is not the only the concern regarding GMOs.

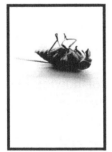

In 1985, Bayer CropScience, a Belgium company, was first to develop engineered tobacco plants using a product called Bacillus thuringiensis (Bt) as an affective insecticide. When an insect eats a plant treated with Bt, it causes pores, lesions, and tears in the stomach. Bt also has an anticoagulant chemical that blocks the absorbtion of vitamin K inhibiting the body's ability to clot causing the insect to bleed to death.

Ten years later the FDA approved the usages of Bt on potato crops grown in the US. Additionally, Monsanto made the discovery that the pink bull-worms were resistant to Bt usage on the cotton crops in India which caused an infestation ruining thousands of crops for several years.

Today, India is the largest producer of cotton in the world. Over 80% of the cotton-growing areas use GMOs and Bt. There is a lot of controversy over the use of Bt cotton. Farmers are being forced to buy only GMO seeds and not allowed to keep any seeds from one season to another. This way the costs to grow cotton is regulated by the seed companies (primarily Monsanto) which keep the prices so high that many farmers have gone bankrupt and/or committed suicide.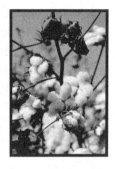

"Compared to a spray application of Bacillus thuringiensis, a genetically- modified crop produces Bt at concentrations thousands of times higher. After Bt is sprayed, it breaks down fairly soon. With a genetically-modified crop, the Bt survives in the plant tissue long after harvest," states Micheal Fields of Agricultural Institute. This includes the cotton seed which is pressed to produce cotton seed oil. (Next time you look at a food label, notice have many food products contain cotton seed oil) Furthermore, because Bt is concentrated in the plant's root system, it winds up in the soil and waterways.

Fields goes on to say, "Now the Bt toxin is showing up in the bloodstream of humans. Researchers in Canada looked for signs of the bio-pesticide in the blood of pregnant and non-pregnant women. A study published in Reproductive Toxicology in February 2011 found the Bt toxin in 93% of maternal blood samples, 80% of fetal blood samples, and 69% of non-pregnant women blood samples."

The EPA claims that Bt is safe because it only affects certain insects but a new study in 2012 shows that Bt causes tears in human cells as well as insects. Many scientists and professionals who feel it necessary to speak out believe this explains why there has been an acceleration in the past few years of gastrointestinal diseases.

Garry Gordon, MD, DO, author of *The Chelation Answer*, states, "if Bt is causing an increase propensity for our intestines to become permeable and leaky or food to be presented to our bloodstream in a premature fashion, the havoc it will cause will be across the entire spectrum of disease; from premature aging, Alzheimer's to Parkinson's to Autism to cancer to asthma."

An interesting occurrence using Bt is that the specific insects that it is designed to target are becoming resistant to the chemical. So many farmers are facing an infestation of insects instead of a decrease infestation. Also, Bt is suspected of killing lady bugs, butterflies, bees, and other insects beneficial to a healthy environment.

So why are there **no warning labels** on products of the awful side affects of GMOs and Bt? Well, Dr Oz asked the same question on one of his shows. He invited three experts to discuss GMOs, as well as, Monsanto. Monsanto declined but offered this response, "Requiring labeling for ingredients that don't pose a health issue would undermine both the labeling laws and the consumer confidence."

Wow! I don't know about you, but *my confidence* in Monsanto or any other company manufacturing and *supporting the use of GMOs and Bt is already undermined! I do not believe they have my best interest at heart.*

So how else is "man" changing the food we eat?

Recombinant bovine growth hormone (rBGH) or recombinant bovine somatotropin (rBST) refers to bovine growth hormone that is injected into lactating cows which is artificially made in a lab using genetic technology to stimulate milk production.

However, a side effect of this hormone is udder inflammation called mastics. Huge amounts of antibiotics are given to control the spread of infection. Puss along with the hormone and antibiotics are passed into the milk and ultimately to the consumer. *(that's you, me, and our children - ick!)*

Many countries in Europe and Canada have banned the use of rBHG and rBST but the FDA still approves the use. "Got Milk" has a whole new meaning - right?

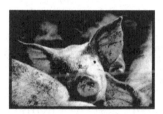 The chicken and hog industries are using hormones as well as inhumane living environments for the animals, housing them in cages and pens where the animals can barely move and constantly standing in fecal material.

Additionally, with the rise in demand of fish protein, the farm fishing industry is booming. Marine Harvest, the world's largest fish farmer, owns 92% of the salmon farming in British Colombia, Canada.

All sorts of problems are surfacing as fish farming is taking over and running the wild salmon fishing industry out of business. Ever since farmed fish were introduced, more and more wild salmon are disappearing. Partly because the escaped farm fish compete for food sources and partly due to lice and disease.

Alexandra Morton, Biologist for the Raincoast Research Society, says, "In the normal environment, little salmon shouldn't have any lice - very, very rare to find any lice on them at all. But what is happening now is these little fish meet these huge populations of farmed salmon and as these little guys go by, they are going through a cloud of baby lice. Theses little fish have to swim near the shore and the fish farms are tied to the shore so they get infected with lice." She believes that 60% of those fish exposed to 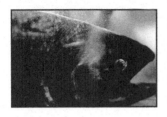 lice, will prematurely die. The rest will infect other wild salmon.

The fish pen enclosures can have as many as 50,000 individuals in each enclosure - allowing each fish the space the size of a bathtub. Many fish go blind and become insane attacking each other and rubbing against the side of the pen causing injuries. And the farmed trout pens sometimes hold up to three times that amount of fish.

Fish pellets are laden with chemicals and antibiotics that lead to the cause of the higher PCB and dioxin contamination levels which are many times higher than the already-dangerous levels found in wild salmon.

A study was done by the Institute for Health and the Environment - University of Albany, showing exceedingly high levels of contaminants in farmed salmon:

        PCBs - banned in the US in 1976 because it causes caner

        Dioxins - causes cancer, reproductive and developmental
            effects, alters immune function, and toxic to fetal
            endocrine system

        Toxaphene - banned in 1982 for damage to the liver,
            kidneys, nervous system, and adrenal glands

        Dieldrin - banned in 1974 because it is considered a
            carcinogen by the EPA

Furthermore, it is stated that, "The authors concluded that concentrations of several cancer-causing substances are high enough to suggest that consumers should consider restricting their consumption of farmed salmon. In most cases, consumption of more than one meal of farmed salmon per month could pose unacceptable cancer risks according to U.S. Environmental Protection Agency (EPA) methods for calculating fish consumption advisories."

PBS did a *Newshour* piece on the farmed salmon and Lee Hochberg said, "The study in Science magazine was the largest of its kind. It analyzed two tons of farm salmon for 14 different organic contaminants, including PCBs and dioxins, which can cause cancer. It compared levels in those fish from more than 50 farms in eight regions of the world, to contamination levels found in wild salmon. It concluded farm salmon had ten times the level of contaminants of wild salmon. And eating farm salmon can increase one's risk of getting cancer."

Did you know that most of the farmed salmon in the US comes from Chile, not BC, Canada? There had never been salmon along the Patagonia coast until the open cage fish farming industry exploded along the coastline.

In an article written by Dan Shapley of The Daily Green called, *The Problem with Farmed Atlantic Salmon,* states, "Prompted by Oceana, Chile has revealed that its fish farms use hundreds of times more antibiotics than Norway, the world's leading producer of farmed salmon, according to a report in the New York Times. Chile provides most of the farmed salmon available on the U.S. market, according to the Environmental Defense Fund, which had already labeled farmed Atlantic salmon as an 'eco-worst' choice at the fish market."

In 2007, the fish pens were infested with a lethal microbe called infectious salmon anemia (ISA), a flu-like virus that wiped out millions of fish. The carcases of the dead diseased fish contaminated the ecosystem of the whole area for miles and scientists believe it may take ten years for the marine life to recover. This happened in Ireland, Scotland, and Norway as well.

Well, the big fish farmers were not willing to wait that long so they rebuilt the pens and came up with a remedy - ***more chemicals*** - more antibiotics to kill the viruses and infections. Although this does not answer the lice epidemic issue. **Oh yes, we consume these lice when eating farmed fish** - not just salmon, but all farmed fish like tilapia, trout, catfish, sole, and more.

In addition, farmed salmon is grayish white in color which means more added chemicals, synthetic pigment replacements, are mixed into the fish food pellets to produce the pink colored flesh, albeit not the bright pink color as that of wild salmon. And many people liken the texture to stiff smashed potatoes.

OK, that's about farmed salmon, what about genetically engineered salmon - that's right, another example of "man" playing God again. This "man-made fish" has not been approved for mass producing yet so there is still time to do something before it's too late.

This *Frankenfish*, as it has been aptly coined, grows twice as fast as farmed salmon and poses an even greater threat to the extinction of the wild salmon population than farmed fish.

The Center For Food Safety says, "GE fish pose serious risks to wild salmon and our marine environment. Each year millions of farmed salmon escape from open water net pens, out competing wild salmon for resources. To make matters worse, GE fish would cause genetic pollution. Studies show that the release of just 60 GE fish into a wild salmon population of 60,000 would lead to the extinction of the wild fish in less that 40 fish generations."

Whether this would happen purposely or accidentally, once the introduction began, the extinction of wild populations cannot be stopped. Although the word *genocide* did not exists before 1944 and applies to humans, I believe this is exactly what would happen to all native fish world wide. As to date, these "mini-god" scientists are developing 35 genetically engineered species of fish.

"The genes engineered in these experimental fish come from a variety of organisms, including other fish, coral, mice, bacteria, and even humans", states the Center For Food Safety.

It is believed that these GE fish are more prone to anti-resistant viruses allowing new infections thus requiring even more antibiotics than farmed fish which currently receive more per pound than cattle. And *just like the beef that is eaten, these chemicals will be transfered to the consumer.*

Since the FDA does not do any of its own testing, it relies on the data given to it by the same sources that are promoting GE fish. This is all new technology without any long-term studies. So if this "new" fish should appear on the grocery shelves, there is no requirement to label the fish as anything other than farmed fish - meaning the public would never know if it is GE fish or not. I applaud stores like Trader Joe's, Aldi, Whole Foods, Marsh, and hopefully others who say they will not put GE fish on their shelves.

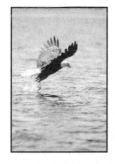

And what about the effects to the other marine life, animals, and birds that depend on the fish for survival? It has been proven that the GE fish are lower in Omega 3 and Omega 6 which would make a huge impact of the diets of these other creatures, let alone humans. And then add all of the chemicals, antibiotics, and waste pollutions as well. I think it spells disaster!!!

Do you feel a little overwhelmed with all this information? Do you feel like there is nothing you can do because you are just one person? Well, I unequivocally believe that what you do right now will change your life and yes, one person can make a difference...

You can choose!

You can choose to eat organic and real natural foods right now. But...............I think I hear some buts...

but is costs too much

What do you think it is costing you health wise? How many times do you go to the doctor's office (ch-ching) and the pharmacy to get pills for what ails you? (ch-ching) And there's all those co-pays and expenses not covered by your insurance if you have it; if you don't have insurance - what does that cost you? (ch-ching...ch-ching). Over 50% of US bankruptcies are due to medical expenses.

And I'll admit, organic food items do cost more than conventionally grown and GMOs foods but the organic food is full of nutrition that satisfies your body's needs so you eat less and get healthier. **Non-organic food is lifeless and dead** - it is full of carbohydrates, fats, sugars, and chemicals.

but it takes too much time to shop for organic foods

Unless you live out in the sticks, there are organic stores in virtually every city and town. Also, you can order organic food Online and have it delivered to your doorstep.

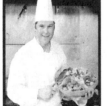

but I eat out a lot

More and more restaurants are offering organic food choices. If you don't see any, ask for it and ask if the food they do serve is GMO or farmed fish. If you are a regular customer, send a letter to the owner or manager asking that organic food choices be added to their menu. Organically grown food is exactly how nature intended food to be. It is grown in rich soil that contain trace minerals and probiotics for healthy, nutritional plants.

Organic farmers use no synthetic fertilizers, pesticides or growth enhancers (no chemicals) that contaminate the soil, air and water. Organic matter in the soil retains water which provides better conservation of valuable clean water during the drier seasons. And because there are no chemicals that filter through the water into the water tables, it doesn't pollute our streams, lakes, and oceans.

Instead, farmers enrich the soil with compost, manure, and plant coverings. Crops are rotated often as means of adding nutrients and minerals back into the soil. Farmers also disperse beneficial insects, like ladybugs, to control the harmful insect pests and plant flowers, like chrysanthemums, to repel certain bugs.

In the US, local, state and federal health standards are required of organic farmers to follow for production. Also, farmers must adhere to strict regulations regarding the way they build soil fertility. Organic food production has the strictest regulations of any agricultural production in the US.

Organic farmers use no GMOs, clones, or seeds. The USDA Organic Rule states that "The use of genetically engineered organisms and their products are prohibited in any form or at any stage in organic production, processing or handling." They close-ly monitor air-born cross pollination of their crops to ensure their crops remain purely organic.

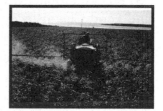

Conventionally grown plants are not the same as organic. Although they are not genetically engineered, convention plants are grown using chemical fertil-izers, herbicides, pesticides, and/or color enhancers. Mistakenly, many people assume that vegetables sold at the farmers market are organic simply because they were grown locally. The pro-duce is more than likely conventionally grown unknowingly from GMO seeds along with chemicals fertilizers and pesticides.

Over the years there have been several debates whether organic foods are healthier than conventional grown foods. There is now scientific data to prove organic is better for you.

The reason these foods are more nutritional is the rich soil and natural growing time frame. "With organic methods, the nitrogen present in composted soil is released slowly and therefore plants grow at a normal rate, with their nutrients in balance. Vegetables fertilized with conventional fertilizers grow very rapidly and allocate less energy to develop nutrients," says lead author of a study, Alyson Mitchell, Ph.D., an associate professor of food science and technology at the University of California, Davis.

In 2008, over 100 studies were preformed by the Organic Center comparing the nutritional quality of organic verses conventional grown foods and found the organic foods to have far more nutritional values.

Marissa Lippert, M.S., R.D., author for an article in Eating Well magazine, states, "As for nutrients, in 2007 a study out of Newcastle University in the United Kingdom reported that organic produce boasted up to 40 percent higher levels of some nutrients (including vitamin C, zinc and iron) than its conventional counterparts. Additionally, a 2003 study in the Journal of Agricultural and Food Chemistry found that organically grown berries and corn contained 58 percent more polyphenols—antioxidants that help prevent cardiovascular disease—and up to 52 percent higher levels of vitamin C than those conventionally grown."

As far as eating meat, I'm not a champion of this. But if you choose to consume meat, please choose organically raised animals.

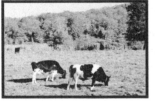

Organically raised animals are not allowed to eat GMO foods. They graze on grasses and are fed supplemental vegetarian feed that is far more nutritious than agriculturally grown feed. Also, no ground-up animal byproducts are given to organic animals causing bovine spongiform encephalopathy, aka mad cow disease, which can be transfered to humans.

Organic farmed animals are ethically raised in open-air fields and graze naturally compared to the inhumane practices of mega farms that keep the animals in pens their whole lives forcing them to stand in manure up to their knees causing bacterial infections and disease. Also, organic farmers use the manure to fertilize the fields instead of polluting the land, water, and air.

Antibiotics, the bovine human growth hormone (rbGH), and/or other artificial drugs are never given to organic farm animals. If you looked at the face of an organically raised cow, you will not see mucus running down its nose as you do in penned animals.

Intensive swine farming is as bad as the cattle industry. The pigs are kept in cramped quarters and treated very cruelly. "Piglets can be subjected to castration, tail docking to reduce tail biting, teeth clipping (to reduce injuring their mother's nipples), and earmarking and tattooing for litter identification. Treatments are usually made without pain killers. Weak runts may be slain shortly after birth. Injections with a high availability iron solution often are given, as sow's milk is low in iron. The docking due to tail biting is a common practice in intensive rearing facilities as animals in that environment are more prone to increased levels of aggression and instability," stated by Wikipedia.

Even though some states have laws that require pigs to be stunned before slaughtering, the practice is not often used leaving the animals to suffer great pain and suffering before death.

"Chickens are arguably the most abused animal on the planet. In the United States, more than 7 billion chickens are killed for their flesh each year, and 452 million hens are used for their eggs. Ninety-nine percent of these animals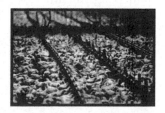

spend their lives in total confinement—from the moment they hatch until the day they are killed," according to an article by People for the Ethical Treatment of Animals (PETA).

The PETA article called, *Chickens Used For Food*, goes on the state, "Chickens raised for their flesh, called "broilers" by the chicken industry, spend their entire lives in filthy sheds with tens of thousands of other birds, where intense crowding and confinement lead to outbreaks of disease. They are bred and drugged to grow so large so quickly that their legs and organs can't keep up, making heart attacks, organ failure, and crippling leg deformities common. Many become crippled under their own weight and eventually die because they can't reach the water nozzles. When they are only 6 or 7 weeks old, they are crammed into cages and trucked to slaughter."

The laying hens are crammed into wire cages and forced to defecate on each other. Their beaks are cut off so they won't peck at each other. When they no longer can lay eggs, they are slaughtered along with all other male born chicks.

Unfortunately this type of farming is happening to other foul as well.

When industrial farmed animals are bred and killed under such horrific conditions, the animal produces adrenaline and other major stress hormones such as cortisol hormone, epinephrine and nor-epinephrine. This remains in the flesh causing the entire metabolic process to change. Lactic acid floods the muscle tissues and changes the meat's pH level, causing decomposition which significantly decreases the quality of the meat.

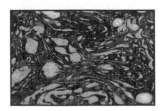

To make things worse, industrial farms are to blame for 80% of the global deforestation, use 70% more energy to produce the end products that are less in quality, and the waste from fecal materials and dead carcases pollute our water, air, and land.

"But I'm only one person, how can I make a difference?" you may ask. *By voting with your dollars.* There was a time when the tobacco companies had a strong hold on America but that changed as people, one by one, stood up for what they believed and took action.

When you buy organic products you support the local organic farmers. Most organic farms are small in size compared to the mega industrial farms. They do not get subsidies from the government to make up the cost difference to produce and sell organic foods. Organic foods are more perishable and therefor have a shorter shelf life than the processed items so the foods cannot be shipped long distances and/or held in warehouses.

If your local store does not carry organic items, write them and ask them to stock organic foods. If they already have an organic section, thank the store manager in person and write a letter.

The more you make your voice and choices known, the more you can make a difference. You can change the way you eat, be healthy and able to make informed decisions, as well as, be a good steward to our planet, environment, and all living things on this earth.

poem:

Changes

by
Barbara Wolf

**What I have learned about
water
is to welcome change,
flow when I can,
become snow when I must,
then a mist hovering over Earth,
or in a fog,
snarling traffic,
even an ice cube,
tinkling in your drink.**

The Importance of Water

The average person can survive without food for up to 4 weeks but only 3 to 4 days without water. Why, because our bodies are 60 to 75% water:

brain = 73% water
muscle = 75% water
bone = 22% water
blood = 83% water
liver = 96% water

Water makes up the bulk of our blood, tissues, and lymphatic systems. It carries oxygen, nutrients, waste, enzymes, hormones, and antibodies throughout our entire system. Other vital functions of water are:

- Moisturizes the air in our lungs so oxygen can be absorbed more easily
- Regulates our body temperatures through sweat glands
- Cushions our joints by adding moisture to cartiledge to prevent wear and tear and injuries
- Keeps muscles well hydrated to prevent strains, tears, and injuries
- Aids in digestion so the body can absorb more nutrients
- Flushes toxins out of our body so viruses and bacteria cannot cause illness and disease
- Dissolves calcium and other minerals build-up to prevent kidney stones
- Hydrates organs for optimum performance
- Prevents constipation and reduces colon and bladder cancers
- Hydrations relieves arthritis and inflamed joints
- Prevents migraine headaches
- Decreases depression and chronic fatigue
- Helps with weight loss
- Younger looking skin because it moisturizes skin cells and increases elasticity

"Our energy level is greatly affected by the amount of water we drink. It has been medically proven that just a 5% drop in body fluids will cause a 25% to 30% loss of energy in the average person... a 15% drop in body fluids causing death! Water is what our liver uses to metabolize fat into usable energy. It is estimated that over 80% of our population suffers energy loss due to minor dehydration," according to Dorchester Health.org.

So how do you know if you are dehydrated? Here are some symptoms that you may have experienced:
- Joint, stomach, and back pain
- Headaches - sometimes it feels like your head is in a vise
- Dry skin - scaly, patchy and flaky
- Dark urine - amber in color and sometimes a stronger urine smell
- Fatigue - yawning often and feel like you haven't had enough sleep
- Dry mouth - thirsty and usually one of the last signs of dehydration
- Difficulty in thinking - feel like you're in a fog or haze

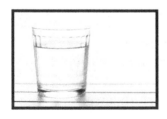

Dehydration usually occurs first thing in the morning. Your body has not had water for 8 to 10 hours. Try drinking a glass of water just before you retire. If you normally have to get up during the night to urinate, that glass of water will not make any difference. Also, instead of reaching for that cup of coffee, drink a glass of water first and wait 10 minutes. You will feel better because your hormones will be activated.

It is recommended that the average person needs to drink eight 8-ounce glasses of water a day. Many people think they are getting their quota of water during the day when they drink coffee, tea, and/or soft drinks, but not so. Tea and coffee are diuretics that actually cause the body to lose water. Additionally, soft drinks contain many chemicals and sugar that the body sees as toxins therefore uses more water and energy to flush them out.

Drinking 8 glasses of water a day may seem like a lot and you feel like you are constantly running to the toilet. Yes, you will at first because your body can't absorb all that water in the beginning.

Think about a potted plant that is in dire need of water. The soil is dry and the plant is limp. When you first pour the water into the pot, it runs down to the bottom leaving the soil just as dry as before. You need to slowly add water to the pot quite often so the soil has a chance to absorb the water. Only then can the plant's roots reap the benefit of the watering. This is like the cells in your body. It may take lots of water over a period of time in order for the cells to start absorbing the water and stay hydrated.

If you prefer cold water, put a pitcher of water in the refrigerator otherwise leave a pitcher on the counter where is it easily available.

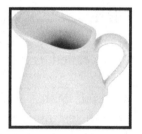

Try adding a slice of lemon to each glass of water. Lemons are a great source of vitamins, minerals, and trace minerals. Here are just a few of the benefits of lemons:

- Taste acidic but are alkalizing in the body - restores the body's pH levels
- Contains vitamin C which helps fight against the negative effectives of viruses and bacterias
- Aids in flushing toxins and dissolves uric acid in the liver
- Increases peristalsis in the bowels and helps with regularity
- Dissolves gallstones
- Contains more potassium than apples or grapes
- Neutralizes free-radicals

- Destroys intestinal worms
- Contains 22 anti-cancer compounds
- Dissolves kidney stones
- Aids in breathing
- Contains vitamin P which strengthens blood vessels

So should you drink tap water or bottled water?

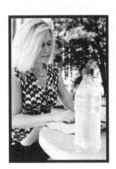

"The labels of the bottled waters do suggest they're special. Some show mountains or polar bears or glaciers. You have to look at the fine print to find out Everest Water is not from Mount Everest. It's from Corpus Christi, Texas. Glacier Clear Water is not from a glacier in Alaska. Its source is tap water from Greeneville, Tenn. Big-selling Dasani and Aquafina are also just reprocessed tap water from cities around the country. One of Aquafina's sources is the Detroit River!" stated John Stossel in 2005 during a piece he did for 20/20 News called, *Is Bottled Water Better Than Tap?*

Federal, State, and City regulations govern tap water. Each month testing is required on most municiple water systems to keep the number of contaminates within the safe levels of the EPA. Although the water coming to your home may be safe to drink, the pipes in your home can change the level amounts. Old homes may have lead, copper, and/or aluminum pipes and the PVC pipes also leach chemicals. If you are concerned, have your water tested and/or use a filter system.

Bottled water does **not** have to meet all of these requirements and the bottles themselves present concerns. "Last summer, a National Institutes of Health (NIH) committee agreed that bisphenol A (BPA), a chemical found in polycarbonate (used to make watercooler jugs, sport-water bottles and other hard plastics, but not PET), may cause neurological and behavioral problems in fetuses, babies and kids. A separate NIH-sponsored panel found that the risk was even greater, saying that adult exposure to BPA likely affects the brain, the female reproductive system and the immune system," according to Janet Majeski Jemmott from Reader's Digest | February 2008.

Additionally Majeski says, "Think twice about the office water-cooler. If it's made of polycarbonate, it has the potential to leach BPA, a chemical that can cause neurological problems, among other things. And have you ever seen anyone actually clean the watercooler? Probably not."

Heat plays a significant role in the amount of leaching into the bottled water. Polyethylene terephthalate bottle, aka 1PET or PETE, release chemicals into the water when exposed to high temperatures. This is really bad because many people leave their water bottles in their cars during the summer time. And the chemical antimony, which is in most plastic bottles, continues to increase its contamination properties with age. Also bottles stored in garages will absorb gas fumes, pesticides and other chemicals in the area.

Additionally, the empty bottles create a huge negative environmental impact. Currently, the US uses 17 million barrels of oil just to produce the bottles. And when emptied, these bottles end up in our land fills, waterways, and oceans. It takes 1000 years for one plastic bottle to decompose.

Instead of botttled water try using a stainless steel canteen - there are some really nice, colorful ones on the market now. Or purchase a reusable bottle that is bisphenol A (BPA) free. Fill the bottles from your tap and/or filter system. Several brands have special filters attached for even cleaner water.

Another little side note on water; in any eating establishment it is best to eliminate ice. This goes for the ice machines in hotels as well. The ice machines use tap water which is OK but the machines themselves are not cleaned very often, if ever. And the glasses/containers may have been filled by someone's unclean bare hands. There have been many independent test findings resulting in high levels of bacteria in ice and water machines.

humor:

PONDERISMS................................

1- I used to eat a lot of natural foods until I learned that most people die of natural causes.

2- There are two kinds of pedestrians . . . The quick and the dead.

3- Life is sexually transmitted.

4- Healthy is merely the slowest possible rate at which one can die.

5- The only difference between a rut and a grave is the depth.

6- Health nuts are going to feel stupid someday, lying in hospitals dying of nothing.

7- Have you noticed since everyone has a cell phone these days no one talks about seeing UFOs like they used to?

8- Whenever I feel blue, I start breathing again.

9- All of us could take a lesson from the weather. It pays no attention to criticism.

10- In the 60's, people took acid to make the world weird. Now the world is weird and people take Prozac to make it normal.

11- How is it one careless match can start a forest fire, but it takes a whole box to start a campfire?

12- Who was the first person to look at a cow and say, 'I think I'll squeeze these dangly things and drink whatever comes out'? Hmmmmm, How about eggs ? . . .

13- If Jimmy cracks corn and no one cares, why is there a song about him?

14- Why does your OB-GYN leave the room when you get undressed if they are going to look up there anyway?

15- If corn oil is made from corn, and vegetable oil is made from vegetables, then what is baby oil made from?

16- Do illiterate people get the full effect of Alphabet Soup?

17- Does pushing the elevator button more than once make it arrive faster?

18- Why doesn't glue stick to the inside of the bottle?

19- Do you ever wonder why you gave me your email address?

Forgivng Yourself

"Forgive yourself for your faults and mistakes and move on." Les Brown said but it sounds a whole lot easier than doing it.

Forgiving yourself is not easy because it is all about you and only you. It's all about exposure. We tell ourselves that we are human just like everyone else on this planet with flaws and imperfections. But we criticize ourselves the most. We've created unrealistic expectations for ourselves by the stories written in our life scripts. We expect more of ourselves because we set up false standards that most of us are never able to meet. Or we wallow in self-loafing by other people's standards or expectations.

At times we may feel that if we forgive ourself, we are getting off the hook or getting away with something, so we feel the need to punish ourself. Unfortunately, the degree of punishment is set by our inner critic who is constantly demanding more and more of us. That inner voice in your head that keeps reading you the riot act for some past event is in control of your life, not the real you.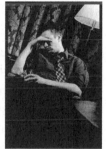

Other times we may feel afraid of loosing our sense of self. Over time, we've created this identity built around our inability to forgive ourself. We're so conditioned to respond in guilt and shame that the fear of forgetting keeps us locked into a past event that replays over and over again.

Forgiveness is not about forgetting an incident, it's about removing the pain associated with the past. You will still have the memory without the negative energy. Unforgiveness burns up so much of your person energy. It keeps you locked in fear, regret, and sadness about something that you can no longer change or redo.

The Law of Attraction is always checking and giving you what you vibrate so if you are constantly thinking unforgiving thoughts toward yourself, that's exactly what you will be given in return. Letting go of the negative and stopping the cycle is forgiveness. First of all you must be willing to be open to your feelings. You must take a look at what is causing the pain. At this point you may not be able to look at an event objectively because there is so much emotion involved. That's OK - you may feel this is uncomfortable and/or risky but keep in mind that *you can't change anything and move into the present if you don't know what is holding you back.*

Opening up may cause some grief. This is not a betrayal; this is acknowledging the loss of a loved one or a part of you that you've hidden from your conscious mind. Many of us may feel that if we ignore something or don't talk about it, it will go away but in reality it only gets buried in our subconscious mind and manifests in emotional and/or physical pain.

Forgiveness is a mindful process - there are no set time frames in which we lighten our load and move on. It is an on-going endeavor that requires compassion and kindness to yourself. Give yourself permission to forgive. When you do, you honor and value yourself. You are worthy of forgiveness - it's the only way to lower your pain and eventually heal.

Taking steps forward will be hard at first but freeing in the end. Don't beat yourself up if you slip and fall back into the your "old" pattern of thinking. That will only reinforce more negative feelings. Focus on what is positive in your life and what it means to be forgiven.

Also, be mindful of allowing yourself to be in situations where you feel helpless or out of control. There may be people around you that you have allowed to hold the power of guilt and shame over you. Once that power is no longer there, it may be threatening to them because the dynamics between you have shifted. That's their own "garbage" to sort through. You do not want to revert back to your old self-sabotaging ways just to satisfy some-one else - you want to be healthy.

Spend some time with yourself and reflect on forgiveness. Give yourself a big hug - you can change your thinking right now and 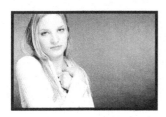 start living in the present. Each time you use the restroom or pass a mirror, look yourself straight in the eyes and say, "**I love you and I forgive you.**" The universe is waiting for those words to respond back to you with more love and forgiveness.

Use these painful experiences to motive you to do something positive - something to give back or make amends. Use your ex-periences to help others so their journey is not as painful.

Take time right now to write down some of the things that you have not forgiven yourself for. Be as specific as possible. Some-times the simple act of committing to paper brings clarity and understanding to an event in our past making it easy to forgive ourself right then. For those deeper hurts, consider if there is some sort of atonement that can be applied. *This is a personal journey and only you can find a solution to your pain.* We will be tapping on some of these issues for homework.

_____

_____

_____

_____

_____

_____

More Balance Exercises

This week you are ready to add a few more balance exercises to your daily routine. So let's start from the beginning.

Remember it is best to find a partner who can help with these exercises by timing you and standing close in case you fall. If that's not possible, count the seconds yourself.

You will need a very sturdy chair that you can hang onto. It's best to do these simple steps barefoot on a hard, flat surface.

Stand and face the back of the chair. Hold onto the back with both hands for balance. If you feel safe to hold on with one hand, turn sideways to the back of the chair.

Round One:

With both feet flat on the floor, raise your toes up off the floor then lower them back to the floor. Now raise your heels off the floor and back down to the floor. Repeat this process 5 times.

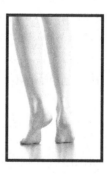

With both feet flat on the floor, roll the sides of your feet in, toward each other and then back. Now roll the sides of your feet to the outside of feet and then back. Repeat this process 5 times.

Round Two:

Lift one foot off the floor while bending the same knee about a 45 degree angle. Start counting (one-one thousand, two-one thousand, etc.) to see how long you are able to balance in this position before you have to put your foot down to regain your balance.

Write down the number in the Balance Worksheet – Eyes Open space on the next page. Repeat the same process two more times. Then total the numbers and divide by 3 to get the average number. Fill in the spaces provided.

Now repeat the exercise using the other leg and fill in the numbers.

This time, close your eyes and perform the same tasks as above. Fill in the numbers on the Balance Worksheet – Eyes Closed on the next pages. Refer back to the Balance-Based Real Age Chart on page 102 to see how much improvement you have made.

Round Three:

Still facing the back of the chair and hanging on with both hands, lift one leg off the floor behind you. Keep your knees straight and do not point your toes. Hold in the position for the count of 10 and then lower your leg back to a standing position. Now do the same with the other leg. Repeat this whole process 5 times.

Round Four:

This time move one of your legs out to the side of your body. Hold to the count of ten and lower your leg back to the standing position. Now change legs and hold it out to your side to the count of 10 and lower it back to the standing position. Repeat this whole process 5 times.

Balance Time Sheet - Eyes Open

Date	1st Set	2nd Set	3rd Set	Total	Average

Balance Time Sheet - Eyes Closed

Date	1st Set	2nd Set	3rd Set	Total	Average

Balance Left & Right Legs Backwards

Date	1st Set	2nd Set	3rd Set	4th Set	5th Set

Balance Left & Right Legs Sideways

Date	1st Set	2nd Set	3rd Set	4th Set	5th Set

Adding More Movements

This week you will be doing the same movements as before and adding a few new ones.

We will start with week 1's program (go to pages 59, 60 and 61) then add week 2's program (go to pages 109 and 110) and now continue with these new movements:

Movement 10:

While still sitting in the chair, keep your hands back in the lap.
Look up to ceiling - Inhale through your nose filling bottom of
      your lungs.
Hold your breath for 2 seconds.
Move your chin down to the chest - Exhale through your mouth.
Turn your head to one side - inhale through your nose filling
      bottom of your lungs.
Hold your breath for 2 seconds.
Return to center of your body - exhale.
Turn your head to the other side - inhale through the nose
      filling bottom of your lungs.
Hold your breath for 2 seconds.
Return to the center of your body - exhale.
Repeat 3 more times.

Movement 11:

Bend your elbows and raise your arms in front of your face.
Bring your forearms together - elbow to elbow, wrist to wrist.
Rise your arms above the head keeping palms together while
      inhaling through the nose filling bottom of your lungs.
Hold your breath for 2 seconds.
Lower your arms to front of your face while exhaling through
      your mouth.
Move your arms back to elbow to elbow, wrist to wrist.

Swing your arms out to the side while inhaling through the
    nose filling the bottom of your lungs.
Hold your breath for 2 seconds.
Keep your arms bent at elbows at shoulder height.
Bring your arms back to center while exhaling through your
    mouth.
Repeat 3 more times.

Fantastic! Now le's do some more tapping.

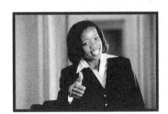

Tapping

By now you probably have noticed some changes in your pain. You may have noticed that new pains are surfacing as others are going away. This is normal. The best way to handle any new areas is to tap on them just as you did with the original pain.

This week we are going to accept more responsibility for pain and add forgiveness in the tapping sessions. Some fears may pop up like:

> I'm not comfortable taking responsibility for something I can't control.
> I'm afraid to take 100% responsibility because it will take a lot of energy, time, and management.
> Having to be responsible for everything in the world doesn't sound realistic.
> Taking responsibility may mean making changes that I'm not ready to do right now.
> I'm not sure why I should forgive when so much time has gone by.
> I'll be doing a loved one a disservice if I forgive myself.
> Nothing can make up for what I did or did not do.

Tap on these feelings. Acknowledge the feelings that are surfacing. It's the only way you will be able to move forward. Add any wordage you want into each tapping session. The following scripts can be adjusted however you feel appropriate because these words are just samples of what to say. **This is for your healing.** Tap on any and all forgiveness needed. The more you do, the more will be shown to you - that means you're starting to tame your pain.

Before we begin, rate your pain level from 0 (meaning no pain) to 10 (meaning excruciating pain) _____. This could still be the original pain or a new one.

Round 1: (see page 69 for chart)

KC = Even though I have this _____
_____(name pain), I completely and
deeply love and honor myself.

HT = This _____

_____(feels like).

EB = This _____(color, name),

SE = In my _____(location).

UE = This _____

_____(feels like)

UN = That makes me so _____

_____(emotion).

CP = I deeply and completely

CB = Love and

UA = Accept myself.

Round 2:

HT = Even though I still have pain, I am open to new
healing ideas

EB = I am open to the idea of taking responsibility for
my healing

SE = I choose to take better care of myself

UE = I choose to make better health choices

UN = I want to stop this pain

CP = This pain that is still bothering me

CB = This _____

(name pain)

UA = That is located _____

(location)

Round 3:

HT = This _____(name) that is
     still there
EB = I hate this _____

          (feels like)

SE = I choose to release all the negative energy I have
     regarding this pain
UE = I choose to release it at the cellular level
UN = I believe my body can heal itself
CP = I give myself permission to heal itself
CB = This pain needs to be gone
UA = I choose to let this pain go

Round 4:

HT = I acknowledge I am responsible for my life
EB = I love and honor myself
SE = I accept myself just as I am right now
UE = I know I am the only person who truly knows
     my pain
UN = Therefore I am the only person who can take
     steps to heal my pain
CP = I can make good choices for myself
CB = I am open to healthy alternative choices
UA = I love myself and will take good care of this body

Round 5:

HT = I now know how bad certain foods are for me
EB = I know I need to make some dietary changes
SE = I want to be healthy and give my body the best
　　　care that I can
UE = I choose to eat a better diet to be healthy again
UN = I am making better choices for myself
CP = I love and honor myself
CB = Eating healthy is one way to having good health
UA = I choose to heal myself at the cellular level by
　　　feeding my body good food

Round 6:

HT = Even though I have this

_____
(name pain)

EB = I know I have to forgive in order
　　　　　to heal
SE = I choose to let go of old scripts that no longer
　　　work for me
UE = These scripts were written when I was younger
UN = These scripts may or may not be true
CP = The stories I tell myself are outdated
CB = I choose to forgive my past
UA = I choose to live in the present

Round 7:

HT = I acknowledge that my past is keeping me in
      pain
EB = This pain from unresolved issues from a long
      time ago in my life
SE = I have hurt myself and I am sorry
UE = I know that forgiveness is for my healing
UN = I want to let go of these negative feelings
CP = This hurt I have caused another person as well
      as myself
CB = I know I am capable of forgiving
UA = I let go of holding onto my negative past

Round 8:

HT = I know I said some hurtful things
EB = I feel this needs to be addressed
SE = I need to acknowledge this hurt
UE = I hurt _____(name person)
UN - I also hurt myself when I said/did those things
CP = I want to forgive myself
CB = I choose to forgive myself
UA = I love and honor myself when I forgive

Round 9:

HT = Forgiving myself for the hurt I have caused others

EB = I have no need to hang onto the guilt I carry associated with this deed

SE = This guilt and anger that prevents me from lowering my pain levels

UE = I release the guilt and anger at the cellular level

UN = I let go of all negative feelings I have

CP = I accept who I am with faults and forgiveness

CB = I forgive myself even if others will not accept my forgiveness

UA = Forgiveness is for my healing only

Round 10:

HT = Forgiving is not forgetting

EB = Forgiving is letting go of the negative energy

SE = I forgive myself that I hurt _____ (name) for doing _____

UE = I deeply and completely love and honor myself

UN = I know I am becoming more and more aware of my behavior

CP = I choose to change my past and live in the present

CB = I choose to heal myself at the cellular level

UA = I deeply and completely love myself

Homework for Week 3

Write down 3 more positive actions that you might like to do. If you didn't accomplish last week's assignment, rewrite it here:

1) _____

2) _____

3) _____

Now pick one to start with. Make a commitment to do it today-there may never be a tomorrow. Write out the steps you need to take, the people you need to contact, and the time-frame that is needed to accomplish the task. Mark it on your calendar and make it a priority. ***Remember, this is a life-changing experience!*** So far what you have been doing to expose yourself to life has not been helpful. Giving yourself permission to get back into life is the path to.......
taming your pain. You can do this!

My first positive lifestyle is _____

In order to do this, I need to arrange _____

_____

_____

The date and time I am able to do this is _____

_____

By signing this, I am fully committed to see this positive action through to completion:

_____

Here is a list of movies/documentaries to watch regarding the food and water industries. You may find some of these objectionable and negative - yes they are. My intention is to really send home the message about the negative energy regarding our food and water. If I left this section out and only wrote about the eating organic, it would not have the same impact - how absolutely vital it is to be made aware of GMOs, farmed fish, and bottled water so you can make a positive change in your diet. These movies, along with the information I presented, are meant to take off the blinders so you can see what is going on behind all the pretty packaging. You do have a choice and you can make a difference not only for your personal self but the planet as well.

I would suggest you watch as many of these as you can this week. They are listed in alphabetical order not order of importance.

Farmagon
Fast Food Nation
Food, Inc.
Food Matters
Forks Over Knives
Meat the Truth
Our Daily Bread
Pig Business
Samsara
Tapped
The Future of Food
The Untold Story of Phsychotropic Drugging
The World According to Monsanto

Complete the following checklist daily:

Activity	Mon	Tue	Wed	Thur	Fri	Sat	Sun
Glorious Day							
Forgiveness							
Ho'opono-pono							
Do-a-Dare-a-Day							
Balance Exercises							
Movements							
Tapping							
Positive Action 1							
Positive Action 2							
Watched Movie							
Grateful Book							

Write down any incites or ahas from this week:

_____

_____

_____

_____

_____

_____

_____

_____

_____

_____

_____

_____

_____

_____

_____

_____

W_{eek} 4

4_{th} K_{not}

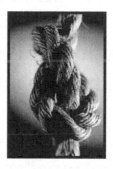

Glorious Day

Congratulations - you've made it to week four!!!

I would like to start out this week just like the previous weeks - sending out positive energy so if it's OK with you, let's do it again before we proceed:

Clap your hands together three times, throw your hands and arms above your head towards the ceiling, and say out loud (the louder the better) **with lots of positive feeling**, 'What a Glorious Day.' Do this two more times (3 times all together).

"Your sense of humor is one of the most powerful tools you have to make certain that your daily mood and emotional state support good health."

Paul E. McGhee, Ph.D.

Laughter

Laughter is the most clearly understood universal expression in the whole world. It doesn't matter what country or nationality you are - you can easily recognize a laugh. Laughter is contagious. It binds people together more than any other emotion.

An article written by Melinda Smith, M.A., and Jeanne Segal, Ph.D. in Help-Guide.org says, "Laughter is a powerful antidote to stress, pain, and conflict. Nothing works faster or more dependably to bring your mind and body back into balance than a good laugh. Humor 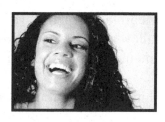 lightens your burdens, inspires hopes, connects you to others, and keeps you grounded, focused, and alert."

Laughter triggers hormonal changes in your body. Endorphins are released into the blood stream making you feel better by relieving tension and stress up to 45 minutes. It also boosts your immune system by sending out antibodies to help fight infection and disease. It improves blood flow and increases oxygen levels which helps protects your heart, gives you more energy, lowers your blood sugar levels, and increases brain activity.

"The focus on the benefits of laughter really began with Norman Cousin's memoir, Anatomy of an Illness. Cousins, who was diagnosed with ankylosing spondylitis, a painful spine condition, found that a diet of comedies, like Marx Brothers films and episodes of Candid Camera, helped him feel better. He said that ten minutes of laughter allowed him two hours of pain-free sleep," in *Give Your Body a Boost -- With Laughter* written by R. Morgan Griffin of webmd.com.

When you laugh your focus is not on your pain so you essentially forget about your pain while you are experiencing something funny. The more you laugh, the more you bring laughter into your life. According to Michael Losier, "The Law of Attraction is always checking and therefor gives you more of what you are vibrating... and laughter is one of the highest vibrational levels you can achieve physically and emotionally."

The remembrance of something funny can linger over a period of time and/or be revisited whenever something you see, hear, or smell that triggers the humorous event. By repeating the same neurological pathways in the brain, the brain changes chemistry allowing you to heal emotional and physical wounds of resentment and anger resulting in more joy and peace in your life.

Laughter is a natural gift of life. Babies are able smile after just a fews weeks and will laugh around one month of age. Laughing makes you look and feel younger. It stretches and contracts the muscles in your face (sometimes all the way down to your stomach) improving circulation and toning muscles.

Practice smiling in the mirror. Just the sight of seeing yourself 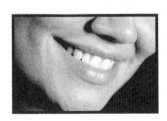 smiling can produce a sense of well being. Smile as often as you can when you pass someone. You may never know how much your smile means to another person - it just may be the only positive acknowledgment they receive all day.

When you hear an individual laugh or a group of people amused by something, curiously ask them what is so funny. If it is a private joke they will say so but many times people are eager to share in the humor. A great ice breaker in a crowd is to ask if anyone had something funny happen to them lately that they would like to share. People will love to share something that gets a laugh.

Children are great sources of humor. Ask them to tell you a joke or riddle (laugh even if it didn't reach your funny bone because the child needs to hear you laugh). Pay attention to their body language as well.

Read funny stories, watch comedies on TV or DVDs, read comic books and jokes on a daily basis. You will be amazed how the impact of humor can raise your mood and immune system. Post funny jokes and/or pictures around your home or office. I like to tape a joke on my bathroom mirror and change it every week or so.

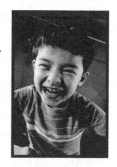

Gather together all those photos you have of your friends and family members making a funny face or doing something hilarious that you captured on your camera. Then put them all together on a display board that you can hang on the wall. Every person who walks by that display will laugh even if they don't know the people.

The mere sight of these items will raise your vibrational levels putting a smile on your face and lessening your pain levels.

Practice finding humor in yourself. When all we do is focus on our pain, we have the propensity to become bitter and cynical toward life. When we are able to laugh at something we said or did, we lighten our own burden of negativism and lessen the reinforcement of guilt and self loafing.

People want to be around us when we can laugh in spite of our pain. Our own higher vibration will draw people to us because they want more of the energy we are putting out.

Conversely, be aware of those who are negative all the time. You may feel drained and depressed by association - you may feel that they bring you down but *actually you have allowed your own vibration to match theirs.* Knowing this, you can either choose to vibrate higher than the other person thereby raising their vibration or choose not to be around them. *Your health depends on the conscious decisions you make.*

A little humor:

Drinking and Driving

I would like to share an experience with you about drinking and driving.

As you well know, some of us have been lucky not to have had brushes with the authorities on our way home from the various social sessions over the years.

A couple of nights ago, I was out for a few drinks with some friends and had a few too many beers and then topped it off with a margarita.

Not a good idea.

Knowing full well I was at least slightly over the limit, I did something I've never done before: I took a taxi home.

Sure enough I passed a police road block but because it was a taxi, they waved it past.

I arrived home safely without incident, which was a real surprise. I have never driven a taxi before and am not sure where I got it.

Freddie

Affirmations and Word Choices

Affirmations are typically short statements or words that you believe, or condition yourself to believe as truth. These statements could be positive or negative; they are words and phrases we tell ourselves over and over again. For our healing to occur, we need to change the negative statements into positive ones. This may also be called positive thinking and/or positive prayer.

The majority of highly successful people credit their achievements to using affirmations. Without them they would still be operating their life by their old life scripts. By placing a high value on the power of the subconscious mind to accept what it is told, successful individuals know that their conscious mind (belief system) will adopt to a new paradigm.

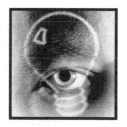

Remember, you are in that top 14% so you have an advantage over the other 86% of the population - *you are already open to making the necessary changes in your lifestyle to lower your pain.* Affirmations will create a life change simply by changing your old life scripts (negative affirmations) that you have accepted as your belief system. Even though your conscious mind wants something different - a new way of behaving - it won't come to fruition if you are still operating under the "old" system of self.

Negative affirmations are self-sabotaging prophecies. It may seem that no matter how hard you try, you keep messing up and repeating the same behavioral patterns that lead to nowhere. This affects all areas of your life whether it is about finances, careers, relationships, etc. If you keep telling yourself that you are not good enough or you don't deserve it, whatever "it" is - that is exactly what you've predicted for your future.

Positive affirmations can and will break that cycle of what was written in your blueprint as a child. A wonderful thing about the subconscious mind is it cannot remember the past - there is no time frame - it only reacts to what it is being told. So by replacing the old running dialog with a new one, the subconscious mind will tell the conscious mind how to behave.

When you start using positive affirmations, your subconscious mind may be resistant because it cannot match the new the new behavior patterns with the old ones. Some of your old scripts have created very deep neurological pathways in the brain causing the subconscious mind to keep going down these same pathways. You may feel like you are yo-yoing back and forth but over time, the positive affirmations will create new pathways. Through repetition these pathways will become deeply embedded in your subconscious mind. When the new pathways are the only ones being activated the old ones will fade away leaving the you with a positive mindset.

Some people may believe that just saying certain words and phrases is nothing more than wishful thinking. And they are right if all you do is mouth the words and expect a miracle to happen. Positive affirmations are not about a-hoping-and-a-wishing something will change. **To create change, a deliberate act with passion and conviction is needed.** The time frame required to make an impact depends on each person's life scripts. The longest and deepest held beliefs may take more time to redirect than newer beliefs. And an individual's openness to change also plays an important role.

Healing begins when we focus on new goals - when **we focus on what we do want** instead of what we don't want (old stories). That brings us right back to the Law of Attraction. Are you beginning to see how our mindset and desires may not be in alignment? Peace and joy occur when our old (not in our best interest) core values are replaced.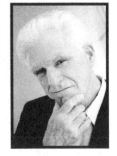

What are some of the benefits of doing positive affirmations?
- reduced stress
- ends cycle of abuse to oneself
- ends self-sabotaging behavior patterns
- creates clearer thinking
- have specific goals
- brings joy and peace
- able to handle obstacles easier
- better relationships
- lessens our over-compensations for false beliefs
- aids in healing old and new wounds
- boosts self confidence
- enhances job performance
- physical ability increased
- less worry and stress

The first thing to do to bring life to your affirmations is to express a desire for what you do want. This needs to be very specific; as an example, you can't just say you want more money - that's way too broad. We all want more money and you have not qualified your affirmation. You need to fine-tune your request like: I make $.50 per hour more in my wages.

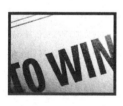
Visualization is a great tool to use with affirmations. Picture in your mind's eye what your new goal looks like. Use all of your senses; smell it, taste it , hear it, feel it, and see yourself already having what you are desiring to accomplish. Bring your affirmation to life in 3-D living color. Make a mental movie of it and let it run through your thoughts day and night.

There are only three requirements for an affirmation to come to fruition: 1) it must be in the present tense - as if you
already have it in your life
2) you must repeat it often
3) say it with emotion and passion

Make your affirmation visible everywhere you can. Write it down on a sticky note and post it on your bathroom mirror, kitchen cupboard, front door, office computer, in your wallet, on your car visor, etc. Another option is to have cards printed off your computer and tack them to your walls where you see them constantly. Add pictures where appropriate. If you come across a great quote that resonates with you, post that as well. Many times using a quote from someone you admire and respect will help convince you that you can accomplish your goals.

Another one of my favorite quotes by Albert Einstein:

"We cannot solve a problem with the same mentality that created it."

Do everything you can to reprogram your subconscious mind. Even if you don't believe what your affirmation says, your subconscious mind does not know the difference between what is true and what is not - it only responds to what it is being told through repetition. The more you use positive affirmations to create change in one area, another will pop up so keep changing.

Write down all the negative statements you make about yourself. The more you pay attention to your self-talk, the more you will begin to see a pattern. Then take each statement and rewrite it in a positive affirmation. At first it may seem awkward but soon you will be able to catch yourself and change your language.

Here are two samples to help you make changes:

Negative Statements	Positive Affirmations
I'm not smart enough	I am intelligent and I am able to do research to find answers
People ignore me and/or act like they can't understand me	I speak clearly so others can understand me

Negative Statements	Positive Affirmations

"Fall in love or fall in hate.
Get inspired or be depressed.
Ace the test or flunk a class.
Make babies or make art.
Speak the truth or lie & cheat.
Dance on tables or sit in the corner.
Life is divine chaos.
Embrace it.
Forgive yourself.
Breathe.
And enjoy the ride."

Solbeam

Media Impact On Your Health

The media impact today has changed dramatically. It can be a great tool for learning about our planet, the heavens, mathematics, science, and art. But when misguided, it has a powerful negative affect on our health and well being.

Marketing people are experts on what makes the public react because it is that reaction that sells products and services. We are led to believe that everything we hear and see is the truth but it's not. *Truth has little to do with sales* - it's all about competition and making money at the risk of the consumer.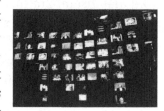

We are told what to wear, how to walk, what to eat, where to live, how to vote, what programs to watch, what music to listen to, what lies are OK as long as they accomplish a certain goal, etc. Even the news is biased and geared toward sensationalism and sponsored advertising.

We are told that it is OK to lie, cheat, steal, and/or have multiple sexual partners. Our role models and heroes are excused from accountability for breaking the laws and yet we still pay money to see them live at an event.

The media has changed the way we communicate with each other. We tend to use TV as a baby sitter where children are left unattended to watch whatever is on the channel at that time. What kind of values are they learning? What ever happened to interacting with each other, playing games, and using life situations as learning lessons so the children can mature into a healthy adults?

Families eat in front of the TV instead of sitting at the table and discussing the day's activities. No one talks to one another and learns how to listen and share in another's experiences.

We have become a nation of over-eaters. We see all these ads for fast food and at the same time are told that we are fat - that only the beautiful skinny people are important. If that's not enough, we have bad breath, body oder, need a face lift or a tummy tuck, or we need the newest and latest widget to make us happy.

Movies are so full of violence and sexual scenes that we are becoming numb to it's affect on our emotional well being. We are told that instant gratification is our birthright and everyone owes us something. We feel we are entitled to all pleasures of life and we are the poor victim if we are denied acquisition whether we earned it or not. If things don't go our way, we act out aggressions instead of using conflict resolution tactics to solve problems. We think it's OK to sue someone for money over things that we should be taking accountability for.

We are addicted to the power of the flowery words that direct our behavior. We hear laughter when someone is hurt so we think we should laugh. When someone is taken advantage of, we root for the offender because he won with the most toys or stepped on the backs of the so called "undeserved" to climb the corporate ladder.

It is said that a child will have seen 200,000 acts of violence by the time they are 18 just from watching TV alone. That's not counting the violent games and what they witness in real life. This leads us right back to the Law of Attraction. Are you starting to get the picture? **Garbage In = Garbage Out**.

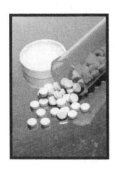 Not only is our emotional health affected but our physical health as well. We are told to take one drug after another to cure whatever ails us. If we are ill, we refuse to change our lifestyle or diet - just give us a pill. We disregard all the side affect warnings by tuning them out or not doing our homework beforehand. We are a nation of addicts on prescription drugs.

Stop the madness - take charge of what you expose yourself to. No one is holding a gun to your head and forcing you to watch certain programs or believe certain ideas. You have a mind that can discern what is positive and good for you and what is not.

Everyone is telling you to be afraid: the news, military, parents, doctors, warning labels, etc. Why? It's not about what's really good for you, it's because **fear sells products and services. Your health is in their hands - not yours.**

You have free will - exercise it - stop being a slave to the remote. Shut off the TV. If you feel you need to be apprised of the global events, watch them Online or read about it in print without the agitating music and visual repeats of devastation and killings.

Be conscious of the programs and movies you watch. Expose yourself to educational, spiritual, inspirational, and/or motivational programs. Watch or listen to a "healthy" comedy (i.e. no abuse or killing) and laugh. These types of media encourage the brain to produce endorphins that make you feel good; allows you to see and appreciate nature and beauty; gives you life lessons to overcome obstacles and adversity; and promotes restful sleep with pleasant dreams. All of these attributes support the body to do what it is designed to do - heal and stay healthy.

Once you remove yourself from the violence, hype, and hardcore selling, you will be more relaxed and energized to do other things. Your curiosity will return and so will your creativity. You will have more mental clarity and be able to make better decisions for yourself because you won't be reaching for the pain medication for headaches and the anti-acids for indigestion after eating snack foods to comfort yourself while watching a scary or violent movie.

Trust me, your life will go on in a much more positive way without game shows, reality shows, series, violent sports events, horror and violent movies, etc. All of which are geared to keep you constantly agitated and in fear and sell products that are harmful. Here is a suggestion list of movies that have no or very little violence - these are in alphabetical order only:

<u>Comedy</u>

Airplane
Back to the Future
Carol Burnett Show
Catch Me If You Can
Coming to America
Crocodile Dundee
Dirty Rotten Scroundrels
Failure to Launch
Fools Gold
Friends
Galaxy Quest
Ghosts of Girlfriends Past
Groundhog Day
Hope Springs
How Do You Know
How to Loose a Guy in 10 Days
I T Crowd
Legally Blond
Little Miss Sunshine
Maid in Manhattan
Men In Trees
Modern Family
Mr. Bean
Mrs. Doughtfire
Murphy Brown
Northern Exposure
One for the Money
Raising Arizona
Sister Act
Spaceballs
Sweet Home Alabama

The Best Exotic Marigold Hotel
The Bounty Hunter
The Full Monty
The Switch
There's Something About Mary
This Means War
Tootsie
When Harry Met Sally

Inspirational/Motivational

A Beautiful Mind
Alive
Amelie
Anna and The King
Apollo 13
Big Fish
Big Miracle
Billy Elliott
Blind Side
Cast Away
Chariots of Fire
Children of Heaven
Coach Carter
Conviction
Das Boot
Dolphin Tale
Eat Pray Love
Erin Brockovich
Eternal Sunshine of the Spotless Mind
Forrest Gump
Frida
Gandhi
Good Will Hunting
Hallmark movies
Hachi: A Dog's Tale

Into the Wild
Jack Rabit Fence
Julie & Julia
King's Speech
Life of Pi
Little Buddha
Lorenzo's Oil
Magnolia
Men of Honor
Mrs. Doubtfire
Mr. Holland's Opus
Miracle
My Left Foot
Norma Rae
Pay It Forward
Philadelphia
Promise Land
Rain Man
Remember The Titans
Rudy
Seabiscuit
Secretariat
Seven Years In Tibet
Soul Surfer
The Field
The Karate Kid
The Last Emperor
The Magic of Belle Isle
The Painted Veil
The Pursuit of Happiness
The Secret
The Straight Story
The World's Fastest Indian
Titanic
Tuesdays With Morrie
What's Eating Gilbert Grape

Forgiving Those Who Have Harmed You

This is the third type of forgiveness. It is the focus of forgiving those who have offended you in some way or manner. There may be several reasons why it may be difficult to forgive that you are not consciously aware of.

You may desire to hang onto your anger as a form of control. The mere act of the offense may have made you feel like a victim, unable to respond, wishing later that you had said or did something to protect yourself. Now you feel that maintaining the anger allows you to redeem yourself.

You may believe the offender does not deserve forgiveness - that he/she needs to be punished for the crime committed. You want to maintain a sense of justice. Or you want to keep them a prisoner of guilt and shame. You desire to balance the hurt feelings - to make the offender feel as bad as you do.

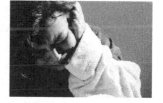

Even if the offender makes an effort to apologies, you may feel that is not enough, you want them to grovel and beg for forgiveness bolstering your own ego with power and control. You may want to prolong the event to teach them a lesson.

Or you may feel that if you forgive you are condoning the offense. That forgiveness lets the criminal off the hook and not take responsibility for his or her behavior and hurt. You may feel by forgiving you are causing an injustice to yourself or you may appear weak to other people close to you.

Even if you feel the crime is so heinous that the criminal does not deserve merit, *forgiveness is the only way to break the cycle of violence.* It is for your well being and happiness - not theirs. Not forgiving colors your existence and interferes with your ability to have a good relationship with someone else. You will remain locked into the past and in time, your negative feelings will fester into bitterness. You will become the prisoner of your own doing by continuing to hold onto your anger. You may feel the world owes you something for all your hurt. ***But it doesn't.***

Forgiveness does not deny the offender's responsibility for the crime - it does not minimize the hurt you are feeling. Holding a grudge may feel like power in the short term but the long term damage causes you to be so wrapped up in the past that there is no room for love and acceptance. You may become depressed and never find pleasure in life. You may become a martyr and victimize yourself over and over again. By defining your life by how you were offended, one day you may realize that nobody wants to share their time with you any more.

Forgiveness sets you free of judgment, revenge, and condemnation. Although you may want the offender to recognize his/her part in hurting you, you may never get an apology or experience sorrow and remorse. Forgiveness does not guarantee reconciliation. The offender may not know of the offense, or don't care that their actions hurt you. Some people are so damaged themselves that they are not capable of understanding what they have done or feel any emotion for their part.

The good news about forgiveness is that it is a trainable skill. It may take some time to go through the grieving and letting go but with practice you can release all those negative feelings simply by focusing on gratitude and kindness.

Forgiveness broadens your perspective on life - life is not just black and white, right or wrong, it is all shades of gray. And eventually through forgiveness, color populates your life again.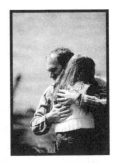

It is for your highest and best interest to forgive - to raise your vibration levels - to be happy again. But what if the offender is still active in your life (husband, wife, child, parent, boss)? And what if they keep hurting you even if you have voiced your feelings to them? You must find a way to keep yourself safe. Communicate with the offender again how his/her behavior hurts you without blame, accusation, and/or attacking. If there is no change in the offender's behavior, it is best that you distance yourself so you can heal and practice forgiveness.

Ask yourself, "What would my life look like without blaming, complaining, self-pity, whining, resentment, anger, depression, and/or bitterness?"

Write down all the hurt feelings and emotions you are still carrying around with you.

Now go back and place a star by every experience that has been helpful and healthy for you to live a peaceful and enjoyable life. I bet you can't find one - not if you are totally honest with yourself.

Last Addition to Movements

This is the last week we are going to add a few new movements to the routine. So let's start from the beginning and do the following energy stimulating movements:

1st week: pages 59, 60, 61
2nd week: pages 109, 110
3rd week: pages 163, 164

Movement 12:

Now stand up or remain sitting and hold your arms straight out
    in front of you shoulder height.
Cross your right wrist over your left wrist.
Turn your hands facing each other and interlock your fingers.
Bend your elbows out and bring your hands into your chest and
    hold that position while you.
Cross your right ankle over your left ankle and hold.
Take 2 deep breaths.
Inhale through your nose.
Hold 2 seconds.
Exhale through your mouth.
Unfold hands and ankles.
Switch positions and repeat the process.

13th Movement:

Place your hands in front of you, palms facing each other.
Touch all of your fingers tips of both hands together.
Hold for the count of 4.
Inhale through your nose.
Hold 2 seconds.
Exhale through your mouth.
Lower your hand and place them on your knees.
Close your eyes – hold your head in the normal upright position.

Look down – to the right – up – left – down again (rotating
        your eyes only in a circular motion).
Repeat 3 more times.
Reverse direction.
Repeat this process 4 times.
Open your eyes.

14th Movement:

Bend your right elbow with your hand up towards the ceiling.
Reach across your body.
Touch your right elbow to your raised left knee.
Return back to your body's center.
Raise and move your left elbow across your body.
Touch your right raise knee.
Repeat 3 more rounds.
Relax your hands back into your lap.

15th Movement:

Lower your hands to your sides.
Shake your hands and feet.
Laugh out loud from your belly.
Shake your hands and feet.
Laugh out loud from your belly.
Shake your hands and feet.
Laugh out loud from your belly.
Shake your hands and feet.
Laugh out loud from your belly.

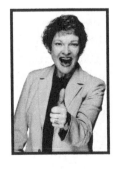

Now you are ready once again to do some
more tapping.

Keep Tapping

Is your body starting to talk to you? Have you noticed some changes along the way? Each time a new pain or issue pops up, fill in the blanks and tap on it. Remember there is no right or wrong way to use the scripts - what's important is that you are consistent in doing the tapping every day.

We will be addressing affirmations and word choices, reducing the negative impact of media hype, and bringing in more laughter and joy into our lives.

Before we begin, rate your pain level from 0 (meaning no pain) to 10 (meaning excruciating pain) _____. This could still be the original pain or a new one.

Round 1: (see page 69 for chart)
KC = Even though I have this _____
          _____(name pain),
          I completely and deeply love and honor myself.
HT = This _____
          _____(feels like).
EB = This _____(color, name),
SF = In my _____(location).
UE = This _____
          _____(feels like)
UN = That makes me so

_____
_____(emotion).

CP = I deeply and completely
CB = Love and
UA = Accept myself

Round 2:

HT = Even though I still have pain, I am open to new ideas

EB = I enjoy learning new ways of doing things

SE = I realize my old habits no longer serve me

UE = I have become very comfortable with my old life style

UN = It's hard to change old habits

CP = I am afraid to make certain changes

CB = It feels awkward to think about my words before I say them

UA = Sometimes I'm not even aware of what comes out of my mouth

Round 3:

HT = I am so tired of this _____(name pain)

EB = I'm not sure if my words and thoughts are keeping me in pain

SE = Perhaps my words and thoughts play a part in my pain

UE = I am open to new thought processes in order to ease my pain levels

UN = I keep replaying old hurtful wounds in my head

CP = I keep saying the same phrases over and over again

CB = What if I change those phrases

UA = What if I forgive in order to change

Round 4:

HT = I deserve to be healthy
EB = I owe it to myself to be pain free
SE = I take responsibility for my well being
UE = I am able to make positive choices for myself
UN = Perhaps the media has had an impact on my life
CP = I sometimes define myself by what I see in the
      media
CB = I am more aware of the negative hype
UA = I completely and deeply love and accept myself
      just as I am right now

Round 5:

HT = Sometimes the media makes my feel less than
EB = It blinds me to all the blessings I have
SE = I choose to monitor and prioritize what I expose
      myself to
UE = To limit the amount of violence around me
UN = I choose to forgive those who have hurt me
CP = The forgiveness is for my healing
CB = Forgiveness brings peace back into my life
UA = With forgiveness I'm able to find joy again

Round 6:

HT = Even though I have this ＿＿＿＿＿＿(name pain)
EB = This ＿＿＿＿＿＿＿＿＿＿＿＿＿＿＿
＿＿＿＿＿＿＿＿＿＿＿＿＿＿＿(feels like).
SE = This ＿＿＿＿＿＿＿＿＿＿＿＿(color, name),
UE = In my ＿＿＿＿＿＿＿＿＿＿＿＿(loca-
tion).
UN = This ＿＿＿＿＿＿＿＿＿＿＿＿＿＿
＿＿＿＿＿＿＿＿＿＿＿＿＿＿＿(feels like)
CP = that makes me so ＿＿＿＿＿＿＿＿＿＿
＿＿＿＿＿＿＿＿＿＿＿＿＿＿＿(emotion).
CB = I deeply and completely
UA = Love and accept myself.

Round 7:

HT = I take full responsibility for my healing
EB = I think about my word choises
SE = I choose to change my negative thoughts and
words to more positive ones
UE = I believe my subcounscious only knows what it
is repeatedly told
UN = I choose to tell it a new story
CP = I choose to forgive and let go of all the anger
and resentment
CB = My life is in my charge
UA = I laugh more and feel joy

Round 8:

HT = Even though I am in the process of making better choices for myself

EB = Old habits are hard to change

SE = What would it look like if I forgive myself when I fall short of my expectations

UE = I give myself permission to fail at times

UN = I find beating myself up is non productive in my healing process

CP = When I laugh I feel lighter

CB = Life is more pleasant

UA = I completely and deeply love and accept myself

Round 9:

HT = I look for ways to bring laughter into my life

EB = I engage in positive activities in order to bring joy and happiness into my life

SE = I like viewing events in a positive manner

UE = It makes me happy when I focus on healthy choices for myself

UN = I enjoy making other people happy as well

CB = When I am positive, other people want to be around me

UA = I completely and deeply love and accept myself

Brain Teasers

See how many question can you answer correctly?

1. Johnny 's mother had three children. The first child was named April. The second child was named May....What was the third child 's name?

2. There is a clerk at the butcher shop, he is five feet ten inches tall and he wears size 13 sneakers....What does he weigh?

3. Before Mt. Everest was discovered, ...what was the highest mountain in the world?

4. How much dirt is there in a hole ...that measures two feet by three feet by four feet?

5. What word in the English Language ...is always spelled incorrectly?

6. Billy was born on December 28th, yet his birthday is always in the summer.....How is this possible?

7. In California , you cannot take a picture of a man with a wooden leg....Why not?

8. If you were running a race, ...and you passed the person in 2nd place, what place would you be in now?

9. Which is correct to say,... "The yolk of the egg are white" or "The yolk of the egg is white"?

10. If a farmer has 5 haystacks in one field and 4 haystacks in the other field,....how many haystacks would he have if he combined them all in another field?

11. A rooster lays an egg at the very top of a slanted roof. Which side is the egg going to roll off on?

12. A completely black dog was strolling down Main street during a total blackout affecting the entire town. Not a single streetlight had been on for hours. As the dog crosses the center of the road a Buick Skylark with 2 broken headlights speeds towards it, but manages to swerve out of the way just in time. How could the driver see the dog to swerve in time?

13. What seven-letter word has hundreds of letters in it?

14. A glass of water with a single ice cube sits on a table. When the ice has completely melted, will the level of the water have increased, decreased or remain unchanged?

15. How far can a dog run into the forest?

The answers are on the next page..........

1. Johnny of course

2. Meat

3. Mt. Everest; it just wasn't discovered yet

4. There is no dirt in a hole

5. Incorrectly

6. Billy lives in the Southern Hemisphere

7. You can 't take pictures with a wooden leg. You need a camera to take pictures

8. You would be in 2nd. Well, you passed the person in second place, not first

9. Neither, the yolk of the egg is yellow

10. One. If he combines all of his haystacks, they all become one big one

11. Neither, roosters don't lay eggs

12. It was during the day

13. Mailbox

14. The water level remains unchanged because the ice cube displaces its own weight. If you're not convinced, read Archimedes' Principle, which states that any floating object displaces its own weight of fluid

15. Halfway. After that it will be running out of the forest

Homework for Week 4

Write down 3 more positive actions that you might like to do. If you didn't accomplish the previous week's assignment, rewrite it here:

1) _____

2) _____

3) _____

Now pick one to start with. Make a commitment to do it today-there may never be a tomorrow. Write out the steps you need to take, the people you need to contact, and the time-frame that is needed to accomplish the task. Mark it on your calendar and make it a priority. ***Remember, this is a life-changing experience!*** So far what you have been doing to expose yourself to life has not been helpful. Giving yourself permission to get back into life is the path to.......
taming your pain. You can do this!

My first positive lifestyle is _____

In order to do this, I need to arrange _____

_____

_____

The date and time I am able to do this is _____

_____

By signing this, I am fully committed to see this positive action through to completion:

_____

Complete the following checklist daily:

Activity	Mon	Tue	Wed	Thur	Fri	Sat	Sun
Glorious Day							
Forgiveness							
Ho'opono-pono							
Do-a-Dare-a-Day							
Balance Exercises							
Movements							
Tapping							
Positive Action 1							
Positive Action 2							
Positive Action 3							
Watched Movie							
Grateful Book							

Write down any funny events, insights, or ahas from this week:

_____

_____

_____

_____

_____

_____

_____

_____

_____

_____

_____

_____

_____

_____

_____

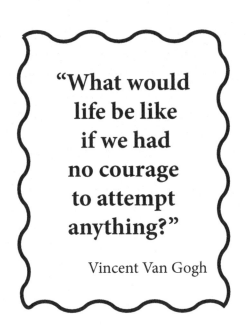

"What would
life be like
if we had
no courage
to attempt
anything?"

Vincent Van Gogh

W_{eek} 5
L_{ast} K_{not}

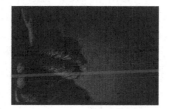

Glorious Day

Congratulations again- you've made it to the fifth and last week!!!

I would like to start out this week just like the previous weeks - sending out positive energy, so let's do it again before we proceed:

Clap your hands together three times, throw your hands and arms above your head towards the ceiling, and say out loud (the louder the better) **with lots of positive feeling**, 'What a Glorious Day.' Do this two more times (3 times all together).

humor:

A Monk's Life

A young monk arrives at the monastery. He is assigned to helping the other monks in copying the old canons and laws of the church by hand. He notices, however, that all of the monks are copying from copies, not from the original manuscript.

So, the new monk goes to the Old Abbot to question this, pointing out that if someone made even a small error in the first copy, it would never be picked up! In fact, that error would be continued in all of the subsequent copies. The head monk, says, "We have been copying from the copies for centuries, but you make a good point, my son."

He goes down into the dark caves underneath the monastery where the original manuscripts are held as archives in a locked vault that hasn't been opened for hundreds of years.

Hours go by and nobody sees the Old Abbot. So, the young monk gets worried and goes down to look for him. He sees him banging his head against the wall and wailing.

We missed the R!"

"We missed the R!"

"We missed the R!"

His forehead is all bloody and bruised and he is crying uncontrollably. The young monk asks the old abbot, "What's wrong, father?"

With a choking voice, the old Abbot replies,

"The word was... CELEBRATE!"

Intention

There is a shift unfolding throughout the world. People are beginning to notice an energy change - that simply by observing something, it is causing a flux around them. More and more humans are open to new experiences and seeing that everything is connected. We live in relationship to everything around us, we are co-creators of our lives. Nothing is static and time is only a human construct.

This energy field that connects all things is called the *Zero Point Field* (aka unified field, matrix, etc.). Every living thing exists because of this field. ***What affects one thing, affects all things.*** A good example of this is the Butterfly Effect. According to Wikipedia, "... the butterfly effect is the sensitive dependence on initial conditions, where a small change at one place in a deterministic nonlinear system can result in large differences to a later state. The name of the effect, coined by Edward Lorenz, is derived from the theoretical example of a hurricane's formation being contingent on whether or not a distant butterfly had flapped its wings several weeks before."

Scientists have proven that on a subatomic level, whatever occurrence happens to one atom, the subatomic particles retain connectivity to all atoms no matter how far they are moved apart. This means that whatever thoughts, actions, and/or words are produced by an individual affect everything else.

Our intention is the energy we put forth, whether positive or negative, that affects a desired outcome. If you desire to lower your pain level, you must intend to lower your pain level. You must focus your thoughts and actions for a specific outcome. You are not-a-leaf-in-the-wind. **You are the co-creator of your life.** You were given the ability to change your thought processes which changes your emotions and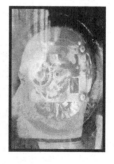

thus, changes your relationship with your body. So align your intentions with your mission in order to start **taming your pain.** Did you know that thoughts form your brain - not the other way around? When we form thoughts, our brain creates neuorpathways. The longer and more emotional the thoughts, the deeper these pathways become. Over time, the thoughts become so entrenched in our brain that we believe them to be the truth but in reality they are only made-up thoughts. These thoughts are not "set in stone", because our brains are living tissue. Our thoughts are malleable, that is, they can be altered, causing new neuropathways to be formed leaving the old, unused ones to cease to function and eventually become nonexistent.

Intentions are affirmations on steroids. An affirmation is a positive statement and intention is putting forth emotional motivation for a specific outcome. The more you practice peak intensity, in other words the more you experience heightened emotions, the more effective you become at obtaining your desires. Again this goes back to the Law of Attraction (the more you focus and/ or put your attention on an outcome, the more you draw it to you).

Sending out intentions works more effectively when you feel happy and healthy. For many of you this is impossible at this time because you have been in pain for so long. Now is the perfect time to be an actor - pretend you are feeling happy and pain-free. Muster up as much emotion as you can. Put on a smile and imagine that you are light and healthy.

Intend with an active expression, not a passive one. Use the present tense only and say, "I am healthy right now" rather than "I will be healthy, or I desire to be healthy, or I have always been healthy". Take a deep breath and feel being healthy in every cell of your being. Taste what that feels like.

Be in a relaxed state (or as much as you can). Even though you are not pain-free at the moment, you are acting as if you truly are with 100% role playing. By using your imagination, you are creating new neuropathways, new belief systems in the brain.

Intention is the power you give yourself for healing. The accelerator to fire-up your connection with the Universe. You were created to be in constant connection with Energy Source but it is your emotional imbalance that is causing you to remain in chronic pain and misery.

All living things emit light. Our thoughts and intentions are the result of the emission of our light. Intend on letting your light shine bright and lower you pain levels.

"The willingness to accept responsibility for our own life is the source from which self-respect springs."

Joan Didion

Personal Boundaries for Healing

Personal boundaries are the guidelines you create that outine the most comfortable areas from which to identify yourself and how you live your life within your life scripts. On one end of the continuum, some people form a very rigid and distinct framework that leaves no room to question their behavior. On the other end, some have no visible lines at all and are constantly being at the mercy of their environment.

There are two types of boundaries that are associated with lowering your pain levels: boundaries concerning your relationship limits with others and boundaries concerning your own limits of behavior.

Relationship Boundaries:

Life is all about relationships whether you've known someone for years or just met, you are in a relationship with that person. Your "old" life scripts determine what kind of relationship you have with others. If someone fits within your belief system then it is more than likely to be a comfortable relationship. But if someone does not fit, strife may occur.

However, over time you may be so conditioned to a certain behavior pattern of those close to you that you have adjusted your own behavior accordingly. You may not even be aware of this occurrence because it has evolved slowly over time. The result is putting your body in constant stress causing an imbalance while the mind has not figured out why.

You may not want to change or rock-the-boat because things are "not really all that bad". But they are - you are in pain - right? You may be thinking that you let someone close to you always have their way - that you are showing that person love. And by letting him/her blur your

217

boundaries, he/she will love you more. Wrong! What this behavior does is undermine love.

If you don't respect yourself, no one else will either. You teach people how to treat you. If you love and honor yourself so will others. On the other hand, if your self-esteem is low others will pick up on your low vibration and ignore or not see your boundaries at all..

Ask yourself, "Is this the kind of person I want to be with? Does this person have my best interest at heart?" If the answer is no don't walk out just yet. Yes, this is an obstacle but it can be overcome. It is up to you to change the tides.

By now I'm confident that you have surmised that your old paradigm is presently not conducive to your health. You are in pain and there is a reason - your body is telling you to make some changes in your lifestyle.

Here's another exercise for you. Block out some time for yourself alone so you are able to focus on your responses:

> Write down each person you interact with.
> How do they make you feel about yourself?
> What do you think their motives are when they say or
>   do something to you?
> Are they doing these things out of mallice or are they
>   behaving out of rote?

If you have any heightened negative energy after writing out your responses, put it aside until you can discharge any resentment and/or anger before continuing on. For the next part, you should be in a non-judgmental place. It will do no good to start blaming either the person in concern or yourself for allowing certain behaviors.

Take a couple of deep breathes. Now write down an action and words you feel comfortable using with each person. *Keep it about how you feel - how it affects you* . Use language like, when this happens, I feel ...Tell them what you want from them and ask for their support. It will be counter productive to attack the other person. Your goal is to change the behavior not irritate or worse, alienate the relationship.

If this new dialog is uncomfortable, practice saying it in the mirror. Look yourself in the eyes and say it with heart-felt sincerity. Keep saying it until you are confident that you can deliver your message without faltering or getting into an argument.

Stick to the script - just the facts about your feelings. The other person may find you accusatory if you say, "you always do this." Instead say something like, "when ____ 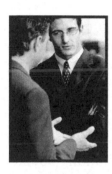 happens, I feel hurt." You want to maintain balance not control. Be open to a new relationship that is flexible - not demanding or rigid. This is a process of discovering what your new life scripts are and how to incorporate them into a new relationship with others. You are setting boundaries where there probably have never been before. You want to have a healthy relationship so you can have a healthy body.

Be patient but do expect a reaction. The reaction may be one of surprise and wanting to make adjustments to better the relationship. Or there may be resistance. After all you have always behaved a certain way and now the other person is taken completely off guard by this new you. If you feel a strong connection with this relationship, seek professional help if the two of you cannot overcome habitual behavior patterns.

However, if the other person is unwilling to support you, be prepared for the alternative - they may fall away. If that happens it was time for both of you to go on other paths. You were never going to raise the negative energy between you two in order to foster your healing. Do not be disparaged, new people will come into your life. They will be attracted to your higher energy vibration of self respect, self esteem, and clear boundaries. Believe in yourself and others will too. You are in that 14% who truly want to start **taming your pain.**

Boundaries For Yourself:

OK, we addressed the issue when others invade or ignore your boundaries but what about those times when you invade or ignore other's boundaries?

Are you the type of person who gets angry quickly over the least little thing or blows everything out of proportion? Are you unable to stop yourself from a compulsive behavior? Do you try to convince everyone that you are right and they are wrong? Do you like offending people just for the fun of it or because it makes you feel more important than them? Do you pat yourself on the back for being able to break the rules and get away with it?

If you answered yes (or partly yes) to any of these questions, you have very wavy or invisible boundaries for your own behaviorial framework. Weak, mushy or non-existent self-limiting boundaries usually mean low self esteem as well. You cover it well by behaving in an outward negative manner. This also creates a lot of stress on your body. Internally your body knows you are

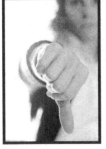

behaving poorly thus producing cortisol and adrenalin (which causes inflammation - and inflammation causes illness and pain).

Take some time and write down those areas where you recognized that you crossed a boundary or were out of control with no boundaries. See if you can decipher the trigger points - you know those buttons that get pushed that catapult you go into those old automatic negative behavior patterns.

When you have identified the specifics, write a new behavior action you intend to exhibit when you are confronted with a situation that initiates a particular reaction. Practice this new script over and over until you feel confident with the outcome. The more you practice this new behavior, the more you will be able to recognize the same old pattern and side step it before it occurs.

Do not judge or beat yourself up for what has happened in the past. *Every moment is an opportunity to create a new experience.*

Perhaps you can find a coach or someone who is willing to work with you. Many years ago my husband and I started the practice of using subtle hand signals when one of us starts to step out of our predetermined bounds. These gestures were mutually agreed upon 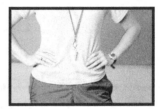 early in our relationship, only used to help each other, and have saved us many times. Also, using a specific hand signal takes the chance of misinterpreting a tone or attitude out of the equation.

Behaving appropriately within your new life scripts makes you feel good about yourself. You don't have to waste time and energy worrying about what you said or what you did to offend someone. You are more relaxed and find enjoyment in life. You will be drawing people to you instead of repelling them. You raise your energy level with your confidence which produces endorphins in your body. More good stuff to lower your pain levels.

"Think twice before
you speak,
because your words
and influence
will plant the seed
of either success
or failure
in the mind
of another.

Napoleon Hill

Your Life Scripts for Others

By now you are familiar with your own life scripts and the power they have with your behavior. Well, the scripts you write for other people in your life are just as powerful. These secondary characters have their own life scripts and are also influenced by your scripts for them - especially if you are in an intimate relationship.

When you think of your spouse or partner as distant and non-caring, you are actually contributing to a self-fulfilling prophecy. When you use words such are gregarious, strong-willed, lazy, smart, cautious, timid, intelligent, etc, you are conditioning that person to accept the labels you have pinned on them and their behavior supports those words.

Masaru Emoto, author of *The Hidden Messages in Water*, scientifically proved the power of words by freezing ice crystals and photographing them. He found that, "water from clear springs 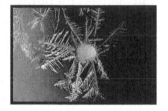 and water that had been exposed to loving words shows brilliant, complex, and colorful snowflake patterns. In contrast, polluted water, or water exposed to negative thoughts, forms incomplete, asymmetrical patterns in dull colors."

He proved that speaking the words as well as taping the written words onto a container of water produced the same results. Emoto explains this, "The written words themselves emit a unique vibration that the water is capable of sensing. Water faithfully mirrors all the vibrations created in the world, and changes these vibrations into a form that can be seen with the human eye." Emoto discovered the **two words, love and gratitude, had the most profound affect on water.**

I was fascinated with Emoto's book and the pictures speak for themselves but I wanted to take it another step further so I bought two potted plants of the same kind. I placed them about three feet apart in the same location and watered them with the same measured amount of liquid. I screamed and yelled at plant #1, calling it all sorts of nasty names. Plant #2 I lovingly cooed over it - telling it how beautiful and healthy it was. Well guess what? After two weeks, plant #1 was showing signs of distress. It was wilting while plant #2 was growing and producing new leaves. (I had to end the experiment at this point because I felt so bad yelling at plant #1 and watching it die at my behavior).

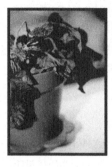 I also did another experiment with two seemingly identical plants. I watered plant #1 with water that had been in the microwave for 30 seconds and then let to cool to room temperature. With plant #2, I used filtered water from the tap. After two weeks plant #1 was almost dead and plant #2 continued to grow.

So think about what this means with regard to our bodies. Emoto states that, "The human body is essentially water, and consciousness is the soul. Methods that help water to flow smoothly are superior to all other medical methods available to us. It's all about keeping the soul in an unpolluted state. Can you imagine what it would be like to have water capable of forming beautiful crystals flowing throughout your entire body? It can happen if you let it."

Thus, your choice of words and thoughts can and do manifest an outcome for other individuals as well as yourself. Think about the energy you are sending out and receiving back while driving your car, communicating with co-workers, watching a sports event, teaching a child a new endeavor, etc.

Take time right now and write out new scripts for those individuals you relate with, especially on a daily basis. You will be pleasantly surprised at how the dynamics change when you do.

A Triumph of the Human Spirit Story

At a fundraising dinner for a school that serves children with learning disabilities, the father of one of the students delivered a speech that would never be forgotten by all who attended.

After extolling the school and its Dedicated staff, he offered a question: "When not interfered with by outside influences, everything nature does, is done with perfection. Yet my son, Shay, cannot learn things as other children do. He cannot understand things as other children do. Where is the natural order of things in my son?" The audience was stilled by the query.

The father continued. "I believe that when a child like Shay, who was mentally and physically disabled comes into the world, an opportunity to realize true human nature presents itself, and it comes in the way other people treat that child."

Then he told the following story:

Shay and I had walked past a park where some boys Shay knew were playing baseball. Shay asked, 'Do you think they'll let me play?' I knew that most of the boys would not want someone like Shay on their team, but as a father I also understood that if my son were allowed to play, it would give him a much-needed sense of belonging and some confidence to be accepted by others in spite of his handicaps.

I approached one of the boys on the field and asked (not expecting much) if Shay could play.. The boy looked around for guidance and said, 'We're losing by six runs and the game is in the eighth inning. I guess he can be on our team and we'll try to put him in to bat in the ninth inning.' Shay struggled over to the team's bench and, with a broad smile, put on a team shirt. I watched with a small tear in my eye and warmth in my heart.

The boys saw my joy at my son being accepted.

In the bottom of the eighth inning, Shay's team scored a few runs but was still behind by three. In the top of the ninth inning, Shay put on a glove and played in the right field. Even though no hits came his way, he was obviously ecstatic just to be in the game and on the field, grinning from ear to ear as I waved to him from the stands.

In the bottom of the ninth inning, Shay's team scored again. Now, with two outs and the bases loaded, the potential winning run was on base and Shay was scheduled to be next at bat. At this juncture, do they let Shay bat and give away their chance to win the game? Surprisingly, Shay was given the bat.

Everyone knew that a hit was all but impossible because Shay didn't even know how to hold the bat properly, much less connect with the ball. However, as Shay stepped up to the Plate, the pitcher, recognizing that the other team was putting winning aside for this moment in Shay's life, moved in a few steps to lob the ball in softly so Shay could at least make contact.

The first pitch came and Shay swung clumsily and missed. The pitcher again took a few steps forward to toss the ball softly towards Shay. As the pitch came in, Shay swung at the ball and hit a slow ground ball right back to the pitcher. The game would now be over.

The pitcher picked up the soft grounder and could have easily thrown the ball to the first baseman. Shay would have been out and that would have been the end of the game. Instead, the pitcher threw the ball right over the first baseman's head, out of reach of all team mates.

Everyone from the stands and both teams started yelling, 'Shay, run to first! Run to first!' Never in his life had Shay ever run that far, but he made it to first base. He scampered down the baseline, wide-eyed and startled.

Everyone yelled, 'Run to second, run to second!' Catching his breath, Shay awkwardly ran towards second, gleaming and struggling to make it to the base. By the time Shay rounded towards second base, the right fielder had the ball. The smallest guy on their team who now had his first chance to be the hero for his team.

He could have thrown the ball to the second-baseman for the tag, but he understood the pitcher's intentions so he, too, intentionally threw the ball high and far over the third-base-man's head. Shay ran toward third base deliriously as the runners ahead of him circled the bases toward home.

All were screaming, 'Shay, Shay, Shay, all the Way Shay.'

Shay reached third base because the opposing shortstop ran to help him by turning him in the direction of third base, and shouted, 'Run to third! Shay, run to third!' As Shay rounded third, the boys from both teams, and the spectators, were on their feet screaming,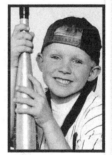

'Shay, run home! Run home!' Shay ran to home, stepped on the plate, and was cheered as the hero who hit the grand slam and won the game for his team.

'That day', said the father softly with tears now rolling down his face, 'the boys from both teams helped bring a piece of true love and humanity into this world'.

Shay didn't make it to another summer. He died that winter, having never forgotten being the hero and making me so happy, and coming home and seeing his Mother tearfully embrace her little hero of the day!

"When we honestly ask ourselves which person in our lives mean the most to us, we often find that it is those who, instead of giving advice, solutions, or cures, have chosen rather to share our pain and touch our wounds with a warm and tender hand. The friend who can be silent with us in a moment of despair or confusion, who can stay with us in an hour of grief and bereavement, who can tolerate not knowing, not curing, not healing and face with us the reality of our powerlessness, that is a friend who cares."

Henri J.M. Nouwen

Loneliness and Social Interaction

Loneliness and aloneness are not the same. Aloneness means a person is without contact from another individual and is quite content both mentally and physically with the situation. If fact, many people seek out time to be alone in order to quiet themselves and rejuvenate. They believe their health depends on those moments alone.

Loneliness, on the other hand, is the perception of being alone, isolated from human contact. A person could feel lonely in an empty apartment, or sitting across the table from their partner, or in a crowd of people.

Typically, people feel lonely because of fear - primarily fear of rejection and/or ridicule from others. Once again we mold our beliefs and perceptions in those early years of life forming the blueprints of our present conditions.

Loneliness is a social pain. Our body is telling us we have a need for connection with another human being just like a hunger pain tells us we need food. All human beings have a basic need to belong. We are social creatures. We are designed to need connections for our body's well being.

Emotional isolation contributes to many health hazards such as:
high blood pressure
depression
heart disease
stroke
memory loss
anti-social behavior
substance abuse
poor diet high in fat
sleep deprivation

fatigue
premature aging
low self-esteem
poor immune system

Many scientific studies have shown that loneliness is dangerous to life. In an article by Paula Spencer Scott titled *The Dangers of Loneliness,* she states, "A 2010 Brigham Young University review of studies involving more than 300,000 people concluded that loneliness is as unhealthy as smoking 15 cigarettes a day or being an alcoholic. In 2012 Archives of Internal Medicine study, older adults who described themselves as lonely had a 56 percent higher risk of developing functional decline (such as losing the ability to walk or climb stairs). They had a 45 percent increase in premature deaths."

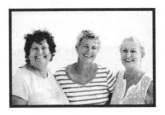 Humans have a legitimate need for social community interaction. Many people have found their depression, headaches, over-eating, body pain, etc. have disappeared as soon as they starting engaging with others.

In another article titled *Why Does Being Lonely Make You Ill* written by Deborah Cohen says, "In 2006, a study of 2,800 women who had beat cancer showed those who had few friends or family were as much as five times more likely to die of their diseases than women with many social contacts." Also she goes on to state, "Psychologists at University of Chicago and Ohio State University have shown than people who are socially isolated develop changes in their immune system, which leads to a condition called chronic inflammation. Short term inflammation is necessary for us to heal after a cut or an infection, but if the inflammation persists in the long-tern, it can contribute towards cardiovascular disease and cancer."

So if you find yourself in a state of loneliness, force yourself to take the initiative to make social contacts. Move past your fears for your own good. Keep in mind that fear simply means:

False Evidence Appearing Real

I know it may be hard to take the first step but take a deep breath and do something to change your situation. Write a list of people and/or things you can do to start getting connected again. Find a club or social group to join. Call people you haven't talked with for ages. Take a dance or craft class.

You can find more ideas for how and where to begin being social again in my book called, *101 Ways To Live Purposely Positive.*

Just like everything in life, loneliness is a choice and your happiness and healing depend on the choices you make right now. *Every moment is a chance to create a new life for yourself.*

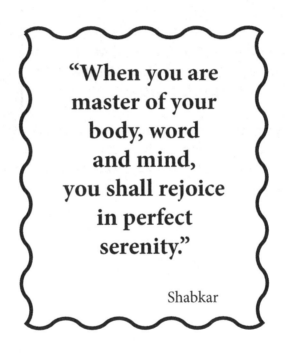

"When you are
master of your
body, word
and mind,
you shall rejoice
in perfect
serenity."

Shabkar

Meditation

Meditation has been practiced for thousands of years. Originally it was used as a means to reach a certain level of consciouness where one could understand the secred and mystical forces of life and eventually obtain enlightenment.

Today, "meditation is considered a type of mind-body complementary medicine. Meditation produces a deep state of relaxation and a tranquil mind. During meditation, you focus your attention and eliminate the stream of jumbled thoughts that may be crowding your mind and causing stress. This process results in enhanced physical and emotional well-being," stated in an article by the Mayo Clinic.

The importance of meditation for **taming your pain** is to calm your mind and body so it can perform healing. When the body is in the Stress Response state to daily events it produces inflammation hormones and when it is in the Relaxation Response state it produces healing hormones.

Thich Nhat Hanh, author of *The Heart of the Buddha's Teaching*, says, "Calming allows us to rest, and resting is a precondition for healing. When animals in the forest get wounded, they find a place to lie down, and they rest completely for many days. They don't think about food or anything. They just rest, and they get the healing they need. When we humans get sick, we just worry! We look for doctors and medicine, but we don't stop. Even when we go to the beach or the mountains for a vacation, we don't rest, and we come back more tired than before. We have to learn to rest."

There are several kinds and ways of meditation. For the purpose of this book, I find guided imagery, aka visualization, to be very conducive to healing. It is best to block out 10 or 15 minutes of time that you won't be disturbed. Pick a place that is pleasing to you like a garden bench, next to the shoreline, in a room with a comfortable chair, or laying on a bed. Some people will insist that

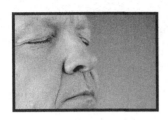

meditation should be performed sitting cross-legged on the floor with your hands held in a certain position. If you find that position pleasing to you then do it, but I find it is more important to be comfortable than look good (who's watching you anyway?).

Some people like to light candles, burn incense, listen to meditation music, ring a bell, or other things to get you in the "right" mood. Whatever helps you let down, then do that also.

The following is my own healing meditation that I use quite often. I would suggest you record your own voice reciting this out loud using as much emotion, imagination, and sincerity when and where needed. You want to be able to listen to this and not read it. Talking in a monotone will only succeed in putting you to sleep or your mind will wonder and loose interest which is not accomplishing the role of this meditation. Get yourself comfortable and then play your recording back when you are ready.

Let's begin by taking a deep breath in through your nose filling the bottom of your lungs, hold one, hold two, and now slowly release your breath through your mouth. Do it again; take a deep breath in through your nose filling the bottom of your lungs, hold one, hold two, and now slowly release your breath through your mouth.

Visualize a ball of light about a foot in diameter. Notice what color it is. Focus your attention on the shades and hues in and throughout this ball of light. (pause talking for a moment)

Start with moving this ball of light to your feet, expanding it to encircle both feet. (pause) Feel it gently start to spin around your ankles, (pause) then up your calves, (pause) and then up to your knees. (pause) Watch it slowly spin around your thighs. (pause) Notice how relaxed and light-feeling your legs have become. (pause talking for a moment)

Next, move the beautiful ball of light up into your groin and hip areas. Let it rest there for a moment while it is spreading positive healing light to all of your lower organs. (pause talking for a moment)

As you move this light up into your abdomen and lower back area, feel a warmth and a slight vibration spreading into your body. (pause talking for a moment)

Picture this colored light getting larger as you move it up your spine into your chest area. Visualize this ball having tiny little effervescent bubbles bouncing in and all around it making you feel light, airy and tingly everywhere it touches. (pause)

Let this awesome sensation spread up into your shoulders. Notice how your shoulders lower and relax as all the tension starts to evaporate. (pause) Then watch the light split as it circles down each arm, making them feel weightless as if floating in mid air. (pause)

Now run this color of light back up your arms and massage your neck and back of the head. (pause) Hear the music of the vibrations as it gently rubs your ears, (pause) relaxes your jaw, (pause) and dances across your forehead - again releasing all tension. (pause) Breathe this beautiful colored light deeply into your lungs, hold one, hold two, now slowly release your breath. Can you feel how every muscle in your body is so relaxed?

Keep the light gently spinning and let it float just above the crown of your head. Notice how bright it has become. Stay there for awhile and watch it turn into a shimmery golden hue. (pause talking for a few moments)

Now imagine sending that golden light rapidly down throughout your entire body; down to the very tips of your fingers and the bottom soles of your feet, flooding every cell with golden healing tingling light. (pause)

Then suck it all back up to the top of your head. Hold it there while it grows and becomes even more intense and brighter again. (pause talking for a few moments)

Again, swoosh it back down through your muscles, bones, organs, tissues - down to the tips of your fingers and the soles of your feet. Feel it flowing through your blood and into every cell in your body. Picture this awesome light vibrating every atom in every cell filling them with golden light and healing energy. (pause talking for a few moments)

Visualize only healthy vibrant living tissue. Visualize your body in perfect balance as it was created to be. Notice how light and airy your entire body feels. Can you see yourself surrounded with golden light? (pause for a few minutes)

Now, take a deep breath in through your nose filling the bottom of your lungs, hold one, hold two, and slowly let it out through your mouth. (pause) Take another deep breath in through your nose filling the bottom of your lungs, hold one, hold two, and slowly let it out through your mouth. (pause)

Make a big smile, hug yourself, and embrace the emotion of gratitude for this healing light.

Say out loud: "Thank you for my healing." (pause)
*   "Thank you for my healing." (pause)*
*   "Thank you for my healing." (pause)*

Now slowly open your eyes and reacquaint yourself with your surroundings. (pause) Carry this golden light with you throughout your day.

Healing Music

Most of us are fully aware of the effects certain music has on our moods - happy, sad, energetic, relaxed, etc. But I would safely say, the majority of us do not know how and why different sounds produce different reactions in our bodies.

Music is a combination of sounds, tones, harmony, and rhythm. Each sound produces a wave of energy that is sent into the air or other mediums. That's why we not only hear sound, but feel it - we physically feel the vibrating molecules hitting our body when expe- 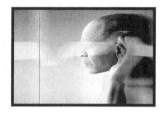 riencing a loud boom or someone close to us is playing a boom-box with a loud sub-woofer.

It has been proven that everything puts out some amount of vibration and the earth itself is vibrating at 8 cycles per second. The human brain is at its peak performance and healthiest state when it also is vibrating at the same cycle rate as the earth even though it is capable of accepting vibrations from 1 to 39 cycles per second. So any vibration below or above 8 cycles per second is putting our brain and body out of balance.

Healing music, aka sound healing, has been known for centuries but it was only reserved for the ancient royalty. It is music that is primarily performed in the alpha range which is the most pleasing to our mind, body, and spirit. When our brains register this vibration they automatically connect with the earth's vibration.

When you change your brain wave frequency to resonate with the earth's frequency, you enhance your body's healing modality causing all of your organs to communicate with each other to work in harmony. Also, the heart is able to regulate at its optimum performance for the total good of the body.

Steven Halpern is a present day pioneer in the healing music industry. When he started composing and making this type of music available to the public, the US government banned his music because "it affected brain waves". But now it is proven that all music affects brain waves. Since then, Halpern has gone on the produce many CDs along with many other artists.

The US military recognized Halpern's music and has been experimenting for the past 30 years using brain wave music. Generals and top officials use alpha-D music to meditate and quiet the mind before making "peace" decisions in order to get into the most effective state of mind. Also, many CEOs and high profile people have incorporated this type of music into their business for themselves as well as their employees.

Additionly, large institutions are studying the healing capabilities of sound and music such as NASA, Drake Medical Center, Keele University in England, the National Naval Medical Center in Bethesda, MD, the National Institute of Health in Wash. DC, and others.

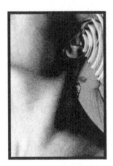

The well known Bulgarian Psychiatrist, Gorgi Lanzanoff, performed several experiments testing the learning capabilities of individuals listening to different types of music and sounds. He discovered *almost super learning abilities of those who listened to Baroque music* (1600 - 1760) of composers like Bach, Vivaldi, Telemann, and Handel, Pachelbel, Purcell, and Scarlatti.

In addition, sound therapy is shifting our health care paradigms. Not only does it calm the body but it increases the blood flow to all areas of our body which increases healing. Many people are finding less pain while listening to alpha sound music. By playing music that has the sound frequencies built into it, it changes the brain wave function which clinically shows a sympathetic response in the brain. Co-ordinating the left and right brain wave activity, called entrainment, reduces stress through relaxation, promoting health.

According to Jeffrey D. Thompson, D.C.,B.F.A. of the Center for Neuroacoustic Research, we are able to prove this because, "Today, with highly sophisticated technological equipment, we can not only observe the functioning of the body and the brain in unprecedented detail, but also measure the changes that take place in the brain and body in different states of consciousness and different states of health."

Here is a graph courtesy of Transparent Corp. showing one of their research study's results:

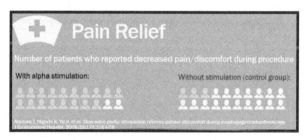

There are several artists who have used alpha brain waves in their music - I highly recommend you purchase one (Steven Halpern's *Deep Alpha* is a Grammy award winner). This type of healing music can be played softly in the background at home and/or work - all you have to do is listen and your brain will start vibrating to the sounds produced.

Thompson also has some very interesting observations. He says, "Experiments with sound have led to some startling revelations. An interesting thing happens when recordings of people speaking are speeded up and slowed down. If these recordings are doubled in speed three times (raising the pitch by three octaves), human speech patterns sound remarkably like birds chirping, When raised in speed by eight octaves, these recordings sound just like crickets chirping. Slowed down from normal speed by three octaves they sound like dolphins and at eight octaves slowed down, sound like the ebb and flow of the ocean.

It is interesting that recordings from the human voice should sound like nature sounds. What happens if we take crick-et sounds and slow them down? They sound like birds chirping. Bird sounds 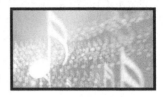 slowed down sound like dolphins, and dolphin sounds slowed down sound like people singing."

As always, mother nature is all around us, part of us, and in us. We are all one. The only separation is that which we manufacture in our minds by our beliefs and by the frequency of our brain waves.

Other Healing Modalities

There are several other healing modalities that I highly recommend you explore. All of these can provide the body with some relief. Since each one of you have your own unique conditions, it is best that you invest some time to experience which method works best for you.

Here are a few practices that you may find to be helpful in breaking the pain cycle so your body can self-heal. By no means is this list exclusive so I encourage you to think outside the box.

Acupuncture:
This is a procedure that involves very fine needles that are placed just under the skin in specific areas on the body, according to the desired outcome, along the body's energy meridians. The ancient Chinese methods have been used for centuries. I highly recommend *Xiapin Song of Qualicare Natural Health Clinic (Bellevue, WA).* She incorporates Chinese herbs in her practice as well.

Acupressure:
This method uses the same meridians as acupuncture without needles. The practitioner uses the hands/fingers to apply pressure to unblock the body's energy for healing.

Art Therapy:
Although this form of healing is primarily used as psychotherapy, many people have discovered physical relief as well. There are many forms of art therapy such as painting, ceramics, sculpturing, sewing, etc.

Biofeedback Therapy:
The patient is taught how to harness specific functions of the brain in order to relax. So when someone is relaxed, there is less pain allowing the body to heal.

Chiropractic:

This practice focuses on the disorders of the musculoskeletal system which affects the nervous system. When we are in pain, we tend to tense our muscles and carry our bodies in awkward positions that can, and often does, pull our bones out of alignment. I have been to many chiropractors and have found the majority of them to perform their craft in an automatic, rote-like, manner which gives little relief over time. In my opinion there are two chiropractors that stand far above the rest: Dr. Eric Lindsell (Columbia, MD) is so gentle and caring. He literally kept me in alignment during my five years in MD. And the one that ***stands above*** all the others is ***Dr. Robert Cummins*** (Cummins Chiropract & Wellness, Bellevue, WA) by helping me prevent many health issues - ***I am positive that I would not be able to live the lifestyle I do today without his ability to keep my body's energy balanced and healthy.***

Dance Therapy:

Therapeutic movements that are designed to lengthen and contract muscle in a fluid manner. It is also mentally relaxing allowing positive energy to occupy the mind instead of pain.

Jin Shin Jyutsu:

This is an ancient oriental Art of harmonizing life energy within the body and is believed to predate Buddha and Moses. The practitioner use his hands as "jumper cables," contacting 26 "safety energy locks" to redirect, or unblock the flow of energy along its pathways.

Massage:

This is the kneading of superficial and deeper layers of muscle and connective tissue using various techniques. By doing so, the blocked energy pathways are opened to allow the body to relax and self heal. I love massages however I have found that a very gently massage for the first couple of times is easier on the body than a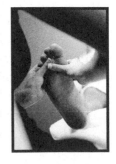

deep tissue massage which may leave you a bit sore the next day or two. I highly recommend *Susan Chasse (Essence of The Sun Bodywork and Massage, Seattle, WA)*

Naturopathic:
A type of medicine that emphasizing prevention, treatment, and optimal health through the use of therapeutic methods and substances that encourage individuals' inherent self-healing process. I cannot think of anyone better than *Dr. McNeill (Bellevue, WA www.ohana.com)* who uses nutrition, vitamin and mineral therapies, herbal therapies, natural hormone replacement, and integrative medicine in her practice.

Physical Therapy:
This is primarily concerned with bodily injuries and disabilities to promote mobility and reasonable functional ability. A licensed professional is able to examine, evaluate, diagnosis and perform techniques using specialized equipment and exercises.

Qi Gong:
Ancient Chinese health care system that integrates physical postures, breathing techniques and focused intention. It is considered a Martial Art practice that promotes healing.

Reflexology:
Involves the physical act of applying pressure to the feet, hands, or ears with specific thumb, finger, and hand techniques using the same meridians channels of energy called zones balancing the energy to various organs throughout the body. I highly recommend *Andrea Day Huber (Seattle, WA)*. Her warm and attentiveness goes beyond a normal sessions.

Reiki:
A Japanese technique for stress reduction and relaxation that also promotes healing by laying on hands to specific areas of the body to allow the "life force energy" to flow into the person.

Swimming Therapy:
Specific techniques and exercises are performed in water, usually a pool. The water provides mild resistance while providing buoyancy as well.

Tai Chi:
A mind-body practice that originated in ancient China. It is a low-impact, weight-bearing, and aerobic -- yet relaxing -- exercise. It is a form of martial art for the purpose of enhancing physical and mental health. Practiced in a variety of styles, tai chi involves slow, gentle movements, deep breathing, and meditation.

Taming Nerve Damage Programs:
A 10-session program designed to lower the pain levels of those who suffer from the debilitating condition called peripheral neuropathy - aka nerve damage. I created this program using the same techniques and activities described in this book plus added more that specifically address nerve damage. Being a sufferer of neuropathy myself, I know have painful this disease can be and there is no conventional medical cure. I have created several packages that can fit your needs. For more information go to: *www.TamingYourPain.com*

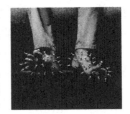

Yoga:
There are several forms of yoga originally from India. They are designed for the physical, mental, and spiritual practices or disciplines to attain a state of permanent peace. In the US, yoga is popular for building bodily strength and stamina. Like any new endeavor, start off slowly and pace yourself.

Sound-Vibrational Energy Healing
& Essential Life Alignment

To me, this is the most powerful thing you can do for yourself. I deliberately saved it for last because I wanted to really stretch your thinking and physical capabilities to start **taming your pain** before I introduced this to you. If I had started off with this topic, you probably would have tossed the book aside and never experienced first hand what **you were (and are) capable** of as far as taking your health into your own hands which is vital.

Although this type of healing is so profound, it defies the logical function of our human brain. Because we cannot see or touch it, it may seem unreal but you can certainly hear the sound and feel the vibration. Think of it as a radio station that only plays static but as soon as you fine tune the frequency, this beautiful music comes forth. Well, that's what a **Sound-Vibrational Energy Healing** sessions can do for you - it fine tunes the body's frequency by raising the vibration of every cell in your body for peak performance. This produces a state of profound relaxation removing stress, chronic pain and illness by releasing the energy blockages so the body can self heal.

Some of the benefits that people have received are: elimination of pain, complete remission of an illness/disease, more energy, focus, bliss, restored health, better balance, clearer thinking, better hearing, and more.

This type of energy healing is simply listening to Tibetan singing bowls being played and following the sound all the way out. The bowls are hand made by monks who say prayers with each hammer stroke and during a session, 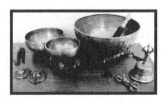 I follow the teachings of Suren Shrestha who grew up in Nepal and was tutored by the monks and now teaches these techniques.

The other part of a **Sound-Vibrational Healing** session is a gift that I have been given. I have the ability to tap into God, Source, Universe, Universal Energy Field (whatever name you are comfortable with) and transfer information, energy and light direct-

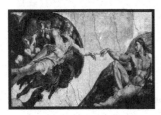

ly to another being and animals. I am simply a connection or conduit, sort of speak for lack of words.

It all came about from the moment I picked up Eric Pearl's book, *The Reconnection: Heal Others Heal Yourself.* My hands started vibrating. Then it started spreading throughout my body. This vibration was very different than the neuropathy "pins and needles" feelings I had previously experienced. As soon as I went on the website I knew something was about to happen - something miraculous. I immediately signed up for the training classes and within two weeks I was completely engulfed into a new way of viewing my life. I witnessed events and healings that were beyond logic, profoundly changing my life and other's lives as well.

Although I was trained by Eric Pearl himself as a practitioner of The Reconnective Healing and The Reconnection, over time, I have developed my own healing style. During a session, my hands are guided over a person's body. I can feel where the energy blockages are and remove the negative energy and I can feel where positive energy needs to be brought in which restores the body's energy balance so it can self heal and energize.

So during a **Sound-Vibrational Energy Healing** session you get the complete healing package - both benefits combined into one session because between the playing of each bowl, I am moving my hands over your body.

If you desire to take another step forward after the healing sessions, I would suggest you have the ***Essential Life Alignment.*** This is an "once-in-a-life-time" - two session process where I

246

trace the meridian lines across your body in a specific pattern which correspond to the Axiatonal grid lines (ley lines) that encircle the earth and universe. **Essential Life Alignment** brings in 'new' axiatonal lines that allows you to tap into the unique vibratory levels and frequencies for healing and, ultimately, for your evolution. These Axiatonal lines are part of an infinite network of intelligence, a parallel-dimensional circulatory system that draws essential life-giving energy for the renewal functions of the human body.

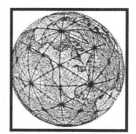

I am confident that **Essential Life Alignment** will take you far beyond taming neuropathy allowing you to experience something so profound that our limiting language cannot adequately describe it. It will give you an understanding that your soul, your inner being, has been so desperately seeking.

If you are so inclined to experience a *Sound-Vibrational Energy Healing and/or Essential Life Alignment* session(s) with me, my practice is called **Taming Your Pain.** For more information go to: **www.TamingYourPain.com.** The sessions can be performed in my office or long distant because there is no time, space or distance that confines energy. I simply ask you to leave your phone on so you can hear the bowls being played while I visualize you on my table. The results are equal.

Each person's experience is unique. Some people are healed instantly but for the majority of people, it takes a few sessions. The body needs time to stay in tune just like physical therapy or other types of treatments. Go to my website and see what kind of packages are offered that best suit your needs and read what others have said about their own personal experience.

Surrender all that
no longer serves you.
Let all that remains
buried in your heart
come to the surface
and be healed.
Let there be space
for new energies
to enter.
A new beginning
transforms darkness
into light.

Author Unknown

Homework for Week 5

It has been said that it takes 24 to 30 days of a deliberate repetitive action to become a habit. Well this week goes beyond that amount of time. The only homework is for you to continue doing the previous homework and keep making progress.

Write your own tapping scripts for all areas in your life. If you feel stuck in your career and/or marriage, tap about it. If you want to start a new endeavor or project, tap about it. Dream about that special vacation you've always wanted to go on, tap about it. Whatever comes to your mind, you can tap about it.

Set the intention for each day by clapping your hands and saying, "What a Glorious Day." Send out that positive energy first thing as you step out of bed. Keep moving. Just because this book is ending doesn't mean you should stop being active. No more excuses.

Be mindful of your boundaries. We all make mistakes so don't focus on the past. It is the present that matters. Make the necessary change in your behavior and keep striving forward. Be mindful of the words and feelings you project towards others. Be a positive force in other people's life scripts. It is not only their future that you are co-creating but yours as well.

Go out and interact with your fellow humans. Loneliness is a choice and one that is not in your best interest. However, if your lifestyle is so chaotic, make time for yourself a priority. Find a place that is special for you to let down and meditate. Your healing depends on allowing your body to relax and balance so it can self heal.

Explore other healing modalities and find one that lifts your soul. I highly recommend *Sound-Vibrational Energy Healing and Essential Life Alignmen* - it is specifically designed for you by your Creator.

Imagine

Imagine if all the tumult of the body were to quiet down, along with all our busy thoughts about earth, sea, and air;

if the very world would stop, and the mind cease thinking about itself, go beyond itself, and be quite still;

if all the fantasies that appear in dreams and imagination would cease, and there be no speech, no sign:

Imagine if all things that are perishable grew still – for if we listen they are saying, "We did not make ourselves; he made us who abides forever" – imagine, then, that they should say this and fall silent, listening to the very voice of him who made them and not to that of his creation;

so that we should hear not his word through the tongues of men, nor the voice of angels, nor the clouds' thunder, nor any symbol, but the very Self which in these things we love, and go beyond ourselves to attain a flash of that eternal wisdom which abides above all things:

And imagine if that moment were to go on and on, leaving behind all other sights and sounds but this one vision which ravishes and absorbs and fixes the beholder in joy; so that the rest of eternal life were like that moment of illumination which leaves us breathless:

Would this not be what is bidden in the scripture, Enter thou into the joy of thy Lord?

Saint Augustine

Conclusion

I am confident that the information presented in this book will open your thinking and your consciousness to new possibilities. Your life, your quality of life, your pain, your well being, are all in your hands and your hands only. No one can make you well, and conversely no one can make you sick, without your consent and participation. Suffering from chronic pain is a repeated pattern of behavior. For some of you that may still be hard to conceptualize but at least the ideas are starting to percolate.

We are merely reflections of all our history, both positive and negative. And we are living systems of emotions, past and present. When we start to recognize these systems and their parts, we can have a conversation with them and we can change the flow towards a new direction. We can assess the past habits of our life for their value and decipher what is working for our highest and best interest; if not, we can discard and replace them with better choices.

If you were able to create a "new" you, what would that look like? I bet there's no place for pain, stress, discord, and/or disease. So if you wouldn't choose pain, then it is a reaction to a behavior - a trigger to some negative experience that is still controlling your present. It is a reactive pattern.

A reactive pattern is the manifestation of the subconscious mind. Every event, every memory, whether we are consciously aware of it or not, is stored in the subconscious mind. It does not judge the events but simply records them. So when witnessing an event, use the conscious mind to discern what emotion you attach to the recordings of the subconscious mind to create a new reality. Choose to move towards, not against, the desires of your heart.

Live with intention and discern between fact and fiction. Unconditional love and gratitude for yourself means even though you are experiencing pain right now, you do not judge or blame yourself for the injury. Be grateful for the moment - knowing you can change it by reprogramming your subconscious mind with intention.

Our brains are designed to learn by visually taking in information all around us; hearing sound and recognizing it with our developed database; and feel sensations with our organs that have memory muscles. The same neuropathways in our brain for learning how to read, write, and do are the same pathways to fight inflammation, infection, and disease in the body.

Taming Your Pain is a choice. And with that choice follows actions. And with actions follows results. It is totally up to you to create the life you want to live. Be a renegade - break out from the norm - take a stand - **believe in yourself!** I believe in you!

Keep doing what you have done for these past weeks. Your new behavior is creating new habits - new positive habits that will change your life and the lives of those around you. Your pain (and lack of pain) will propel you to new horizons and new vistas. Life was meant to be lived not just endured. And lived with a passion that grows deep and strong.

I leave you with love in my heart and one more quote...

"Just look at us. Everything is backwards; everything is upside down. Doctors destroy health, lawyers destroy justice, universities destroy knowledge, governments destroy freedom, the major media destroy information, and religion destroy spirituality."

Michael Ellner

Now is the Time To Wake Up!

For more information go to:

www.TamingYourPain.com

References

1) Kornfield, Jack. A Lamp in the Darkness: Illuminating the Path through Difficult times. Boulder, CO: Sounds True, 2011. Print.

2) "Life Scripts." Life Scripts. N.p., n.d. Web. 01 Apr. 2013.

3) "Littlewood's Law." Wikipedia. Wikimedia Foundation, 28 Feb. 2013. Web. 01 Apr. 2013.

4) "How to follow through/persist with your Goals? - Tony Robbins (part 2)." 5 Feb. 2010. Web. 4 Apr. 2013.

5) "Conscious Life News | Facebook." Facebook. N.p., n.d. Web. 11 Apr. 2013.

6) "Law of Attraction: How to Reset Your Vibe? - Live Interview with Michael Losier in Chicago." YouTube. YouTube, 13 Sept. 2010. Web. 15 Apr. 2013.

7) "The World According To Monsanto." YouTube, 26 Dec. 2008. Web. 16 Apr. 2013.

8) "Genetically Modified Foods in America/Health Documentary." YouTube, 4 Feb. 2013. Web. 16 Apr. 2013.

9) King, Deborah. Truth Heals: What You Hide Can Hurt You. Carlsbad, CA: Hay House, 2009. Print.

10) Emmons, Robert A. Thanks!: How the New Science of Gratitude Can Make You Happier. Boston: Houghton Mifflin, 2007. Print.

11) McCullough, Michael E., Kenneth I. Pargament, and Carl E. Thoresen. Forgiveness: Theory, Research, and Practice. New York: Guilford, 2000. Print.

12) "De-stress, Stress Survey, Well-being, Stress Solutions, Lower Stress, Stress Management Tools, Institute of HeartMath." Institute of HeartMath. N.p., n.d. Web. 18 Apr. 2013.

13) "MUSIC for SOUND HEALING." Music for Sound Healing. N.p., n.d. Web. 19 Apr. 2013.

14) "The Scientific Sound Healing Frontier." Center for Neuoaccoustic.Dr. Jeffrey D. Thompson, D.C., B.F.A. 2011.

15) McCullough, Michael E., Kenneth I. Pargament, and Carl E. Thoresen. Forgiveness: Theory, Research, and Practice. New York: Guilford, 2000. Print.

16) "Bottled Water Vs. Tap Water: Rethink What You Drink." Reader's Digest. N.p., n.d. Web. 21 May 2013.

17) Pearl, Eric. The Reconnection: Heal Others, Heal Yourself. Carlsbad, CA: Hay House, 2001. Print.

18) Emoto, Masaru. The Hidden Messages in Water. Hillsboro, Or.: Beyond Words Pub., 2004. Print.

19) McTaggart, Lynne and Hubbard, Bryan. The Intention Workshop. 2008. Workshop.

20) www.eatingwell.com>food_news_origins/greens_sustainable

21) www.peta.org

22) www.dorchesterhealth.org/water.htm

23) www.abenews.go.com/2020/Health

24) www.naturescountrystore.com/roundup/index.html

25)   www.scienticanerican.com/article.cfm?id=weed-wacking-herbicide-p

26) www.gmo.mercola.com

27) www.youtube.com/watch?v=UD7hQBH4yKw

28) www.albany.edu/ihe/salmonstudy

29) www.pbs.org/newshour/bb/health/jan-june04/salmon_01_26.html

30) www.dailygreen.com/environmental/news/latest/farmed-salmon-47072701

31) www.youtube.com/watch?v=ClgTWTEKiM4

32) www.youtube.com/watch?v=14QK-KtgP18

33) www.michaelfields.org/bacittus-thuringiensus-bug-and-human

34) www.transparentcorp.com/research/alpha-brain-waves.php.

35) www.bbc.co.uk/news/health-21517864

36) www.caring.com/articles/loneliness-and-health

37) www.mayoclinic.com/health/meditation/HQ01070

38) www.getNP.com

39) www.responsibletechnology.com

CPSIA information can be obtained
at www.ICGtesting.com
Printed in the USA
FSOW03n2013021115
12909FS